Morton's Neuroma

Morton's Neuroma

PODIATRIST TURNED
PATIENT: MY OWN JOURNEY

David R Tollafield

A New Foot Pain Series

International readers, please note this book uses British English and terminology

Busypencilcase Communications Ltd

Cover by Dane

ISBN-13: 9781981779284
ISBN-10: 1981779280

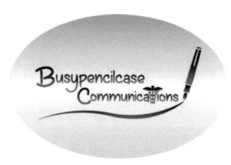

Established 2015

For patients – may we keep you safe and happy, informed and not ignorant for want of the facts.
The Author, 2018

Books by the same author

Podiatry & foot health

**Clinical Skills in Treating the Foot,
Churchill-Livingstone**
With Linda Merriman

Assessment of the Lower Limb, Churchill-Livingstone
With Linda Merriman

Children

<u>as Rob C Blyth</u>

The Story of Cristal Rouge, Xlibris

About the author

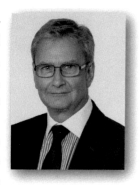

DAVID TOLLAFIELD IS A RETIRED Consultant Podiatric Surgeon and clinical researcher in foot health science. His practise extended over 40 years, with 25 years serving hospitals in the West Midlands.

After qualifying from London's University College Hospital in 1978 he worked for a number of NHS Health Trusts. After gaining his surgical fellowship in 1986 he started his consultant's post in Walsall in 1992, and after 20 years moved to the independent sector where he remained in practice until 2018.

As an examiner and former senior lecturer for undergraduate and postgraduate podiatrists he has written and contributed to several texts on foot health, published a wide range of papers and lectured internationally.

In 2016 he subjected himself to surgery after his own foot pain would not go away. His own patients found this comforting as he shared information about his own experience. Inspired he wrote his first self-help book, although his website. Consultingfootpain.co.uk has been successful for his many patients about specific complaints for some years and still is available to access even though he no longer sees patients.

Table of Contents

About the author · · · · · · · · · · · · · · · · · ix
Foreword ·xvii
Preface · xix
Author's notes · · · · · · · · · · · · · · · · · xxiii
Acknowledgements· · · · · · · · · · · · · · · ·xxv
Quick reference to common
questions ·xxvii

Section 1   How can I recognise a neuroma?
Have I the right diagnosis? · · · · · · · · · · · 1
Introduction · 1
    Signs and symptoms · · · · · · · · · · · · · 2
    What can I do to help myself? · · · · · · 7
    Massage · 7
    Orthotic inlay· · · · · · · · · · · · · · · · · 8
Practical padding for Morton's neuroma· · ·10
    How does the PMP work? · · · · · · · · ·10
    Massage with a squash or tennis
    ball ·14

	Footwear · · · · · · · · · · · · · · · · · · · 16
	Who to see? · · · · · · · · · · · · · · · · · 17
	Pressure (force) plates · · · · · · · · · · · 18
	TIP – help your doctor · · · · · · · · · · 20
	Medical history · · · · · · · · · · · · · · 20
	The examination · · · · · · · · · · · · · · 21
	Diagnosis · · · · · · · · · · · · · · · · · · 22
	Other methods of investigation · · · · 23
	Summary · 24
Section 2	What exactly is a neuroma? · · · · · · · · · 26
	Introduction · · · · · · · · · · · · · · · · · 26
	Key · 28
	Foot types · · · · · · · · · · · · · · · · · 42
	The foot shape · · · · · · · · · · · · · · 43
	Patient experiences · · · · · · · · · · · 45
	A closer look at nerves · · · · · · · · · 46
	Symptoms of neuroma · · · · · · · · · · 51
	Summary · 52
Section 3	What treatment can I expect? · · · · · · · 54
	Introduction · · · · · · · · · · · · · · · · · 54
	Disability · · · · · · · · · · · · · · · · · 54
	Pathway · · · · · · · · · · · · · · · · · 56
	Self-help · · · · · · · · · · · · · · · · · · · 57
	Investigations and consultation · · · · 58
	Conservative active care · · · · · · · · · · · 59
	Injections · · · · · · · · · · · · · · · · · · · 59
	Worries about steroid · · · · · · · · · · · 60
	What other conservative treatments exist? · 62

Invasive procedures · · · · · · · · · · · · · · · 64

    Cryosurgery · · · · · · · · · · · · · · · · · · 64

    Radiofrequency ablation (RFA) · · · · 65

    Cutting the intermetatarsal

    ligament ·67

    Neurectomy ·70

    The scar on the foot · · · · · · · · · · · · ·73

Type of anaesthetic · · · · · · · · · · · · · · · · ·76

    Local anaesthetic (as at the dentist) · · ·76

    Locals anaesthetic assisted with

    sedation (the half-way house) · · · · · ·76

Summary ·79

    More information about steroids · · · ·79

Section 4   Neurectomy. Consent and risks.

Knowing what to expect · · · · · · · · · · · · ·81

Introduction ·81

    Making a decision · · · · · · · · · · · · · · 83

Effects of surgery · · · · · · · · · · · · · · · · · 83

    Risks – being aware before the event · · 85

    What type of problems arise with

    neuroma surgery? · · · · · · · · · · · · · · ·87

    Scary stuff · · · · · · · · · · · · · · · · · · · 94

    Success and failure with

    neurectomies · · · · · · · · · · · · · · · · · 96

    Meeting aims – the clinician's take · · 97

    Failed surgery · · · · · · · · · · · · · · · · · 98

Summary · 99

Section 5   Surgery from the sole of the foot

(plantar approach) · · · · · · · · · · · · · · · ·101

Introduction · 101
    Case study – Brenda · · · · · · · · · · · 101
    Post-operative advice · · · · · · · · · · · 107
Risks and awareness · · · · · · · · · · · · · · · 108
    Case study – Lisa · · · · · · · · · · · · · · 108
Summary · 111
Section 6   Planning and what to expect before
and after a neurectomy · · · · · · · · · · · · · 112
Introduction · 112
    Admission · · · · · · · · · · · · · · · · · · · 113
    A quick reference to admission
    and discharge · · · · · · · · · · · · · · · · · 114
My own nine-month journey · · · · · · · · · 117
    Operation day · · · · · · · · · · · · · · · · · 117
    Into the operating theatre... · · · · · · 118
    Post surgery · · · · · · · · · · · · · · · · · · 121
    Week 1 · 122
    Week 2 · 124
    Week 3 · 126
    Week 4 · 128
    Month 2 · 131
    Month 3 · 135
    Month 4 · 135
    Month 5 · 136
    Month 6 · 136
    Month 9 · 136
What to look for in an infection? · · · · · · 138
Conclusion · 139
Summary · 139

Section 7   Final thoughts and loose ends · · · · · · · ·142

             Introduction ·142

                Factors that make surgery
                successful ·143

                Final analysis · · · · · · · · · · · · · · · ·146

                Orthotic inlays and steroid
                injections ·146

             Opting for surgery · · · · · · · · · · · · · · · ·148

             Author's' Footnotes · · · · · · · · · · · · · · ·151

             Glossary of Terminology · · · · · · · · · · · ·159

Foreword

WILLIAM OSLER (1849-1919) SAID 'THE good physician treats the disease; the great physician treats the patient who has the disease.'

Many clinicians develop diagnostic skills on an ongoing basis throughout their careers. Confusion from false diagnosis can arise, so the information must be accurate to allow for the right type of care. Information should be based on reported evidence and focused on patients' needs

I have known David Tollafield since he was my surgical tutor more than 25 years ago and he is one of the most focused, thorough podiatric surgeons I have met. He has dedicated his career to developing audit processes so that we can be reflective in our practice and provide patients with best evidence.

The internet helps patients form a good knowledge base but the challenge for any clinician arises when offering clear information to support the most appropriate treatment. The information provided in this book is the culmination of a lifetime's career of evidence-based practice merged with personal experience of the condition. When a clinician has the same disease as their patient there is an automatic empathy. There is nothing like reflecting upon the symptoms and experiencing the results of treatment for one's self. This is why this book is so unique.

I doubt this level of information could be bettered. I hope you enjoy the read.

Trevor Prior

Consultant Podiatric Surgeon

Former Dean, Faculty of Podiatric Surgery, College of Podiatry, London

Preface

WHEN IT COMES TO TREATMENT no one wants a hole in their foot. After convalescing from my own surgery I realised that it would make more sense for patients contemplating surgery for Morton's neuroma to have access to a structured book dedicated to the subject without advertising or promotion. This then turned into an A-Z information book to help people who had not yet been treated. While surgery might be the endgame, it must not be assumed that this is the desired direction.

So, why buy my book?
The patient experience or journey needed to be broken down into manageable, bite-size chunks; facts brought together in one place. All specialists, and by that I mean people who offer surgery, will provide information in the form of factsheets. Some are wonderfully presented and, when concise, helpful – but many are woefully brief or too simplistic and omit often needed detail. I believe

patients understand more than we give them credit for, and many facts are obscured by medical jargon. Phrases such as informed choice are considered modern, but deeper down being informed can only happen when everything is fully comprehended.

My decision to emphasise the impact of treatment for Morton's neuroma is related to a greater demand placed on the treating clinician to clarify aspects of treatment, once taken for granted. Healthcare professionals do not intentionally hide facts, but the downsides of care have to be balanced with the benefits.

In describing my own journey, I also looked at the outcome, which is how we professionals view our end results. I set myself five criteria when compiling the book:

* Respect the reader; give lots of information
* Inform and give choices (of treatment, before and after surgery)
* Answer common questions without prejudice
* Explain why treatments do not always work
* Show how critical assessment is achieved

I decided to produce this printed version having launched an e-book. Each section is summarised with key points at the end. Please dip in and out to find the areas most important to you. The quick reference to common questions provides a good place to start. I hope that this book provides confidence in comprehending medical care for Morton's neuroma better.

Thank you for ordering this book.

David R Tollafield, 2018

FCPodS, MSc, BSc, DPodM, FCPM

Author's notes

THIS BOOK CONSISTS OF SEVEN sections, sub-divided for reference with explanations about care supported by information.

I use tips and case note comments with personal observations. The book has been written for the British market (and thus uses British English spelling and terminology), but treatment will vary little in most countries with established healthcare systems.

Where several neuromas exist these can be described as neuromata. Neuromata have many names: Morton's neuroma, metatarsalgia and interdigital neuritis/neuroma. The ball of the foot is associated with the five metatarsal heads upon which we balance. All diagrams used have been simplified, and while they do not represent exact anatomy they are intended to clarify the text.

Orthotic inlay is used in the book to mean an arch support but other terms are used by different professions. Orthoses are commonly made from casts taken as an impression from one foot or both feet, or from computerised impressions. I have used the College of Podiatry[1] database for foot surgery.

'Foot surgeon' or 'surgeon'[2] as used in this book implies a podiatrist trained in foot surgery (a Fellow of College of Podiatry) and called podiatric surgeon; they are trained in medicine but are not medical doctors. Podiatrists qualified to undertake surgery in Scotland may use a different qualification but are registered by the same professional body (HCPC)[3]. Podiatric surgery was established in 1975.

Material used in this book was in date at the time of publication, but references to sites can change without notice. The information published is my own opinion except where a reference is used. All names used in this book have been anonymised.

Author footnotes can be found at the end with the **glossary** for further information. Foot notes are marked but I have chosen not to interrupt the flow of each page with footnotes.

Acknowledgements

I AM INDEBTED TO BOTH lay and professional colleagues, patients and friends who have kindly looked over my manuscript and provided comments and contributions. In particular to Sidney Gibson, Jenny Norton, Lyndon Jones, Trevor Prior, Suzy Speirs, Marius Vintila (Dr), Damian Holdcroft, Steve Picken, Anne Thompson, Nike Akinwale (Dr), Timothy Kilmartin (Dr), those who prefer not to be mentioned and to my anonymous surgeon, I would like to express my gratitude. My thanks go to the College of Podiatry for providing anonymised data and to Selena Class, my enduring editor for minimising my mistakes. Last but by no means least, gratitude to my wife Jill for her tolerance and advice.

This book has no sponsorship. My aim is to inform, promote my profession and offer a different perspective on care while remaining impartial. Products mentioned in this book have been personally used by me as a reference but do not represent the only source.

Quick reference to common questions

What can I do to help myself?   17
Self-help does not make a difference – what next?   23
Who to see?   23
What can I expect (after seeing the doctor)?   24
Why do I feel pain at the end of my toe and not
near the nerve?   33
I experience symptoms in my second/third toe. Is
this Morton's neuroma?   33
What is the Mulder click test?   33
Is a neuroma a tumour?   33
Can neuromas (neuromata) become malignant?   33
If it is not a neuroma, what can it be?   34
Why are women more susceptible to Morton's
neuroma?   35
Why do men suffer if they don't wear tight shoes?   37
My toes are splayed – does this mean anything?   39
What happens to a nerve to make it so painful?   40
What does the interdigital nerve do?   41

Are nerves important? 41

Can we sacrifice sensation? 42

What other conservative treatments exist? 49

Should I select my own operation site? 53

Do I have a choice of anaesthetic? 58

What types of problem arise with neuroma surgery? 64

The risk of scar problems seems low but what of the impact (of plantar incision)? 77

Should we go top or bottom of the foot? 96

How can I recognise a neuroma?
Have I the right diagnosis?

INTRODUCTION

NEUROMA (PRONOUNCED NEW-ROMA)

Getting to the right person to treat you is important. Equally so is making sure you have the right diagnosis for your foot problem. The route to treatment is called a treatment pathway and within this process, over a period of time (timeline) you will engage in a journey of care. Your patient journey hopefully will proceed uneventfully, and at the end you will have succeeded in solving your problem, which in this case we will assume was a neuroma. The end of that journey is expressed in terms of outcome. The outcome[4] can be expressed as aims met, aims partly met or aims not met.

Patients are better informed and educated in health matters partly because of internet access and raised standards of education. The internet, however, provides both good and bad information. Much of the internet functions on advertising and promotion, so phrases like 'best in the country', 'experienced', 'always have success' even '100% success' must be taken with a pinch of salt. Some newspaper articles are written as information but are often glorified adverts that have to be paid for

Every one of us has a responsibility to look after our health, and when embarking on treatment that responsibility is shared with the person treating you. Tips used in these pages are to ensure you are prepared for, and confident about going into, your consultation. My aim is that you achieve the best patient journey right from the start.

This section covers the first part of the patient journey, so if you have reached a professional already you can skip it and go to the end for the summary. Alternatively, you can return to this section later after a consultation, having consulted your general practitioner (GP/family doctor).

Recognition
This is difficult. Why? Your first pain experience won't even register because it is short-lived and easily forgotten.

SIGNS AND SYMPTOMS
Generally, it is accepted that 4-6 time more women suffer from neuromata than men. I will deal with this in Section 2. Pain experienced after walking or exercising is your first indicator that something is not right. The sole may hurt and you may experience an unpleasant or

strange feeling under the ball of your feet, or between the second and third or third and fourth toes.

Your toes may swell or splay. We call this separation 'diastasis'. An electric shock-like sensation in the toe is considered indicative of a nerve-related problem, and is known as a paraesthesia (pronounced paris-theeze-e-ah). The same thing happens in the back when nerves become trapped around the neck and fingers may have that same sensation. Removing a shoe to relieve discomfort is characteristic of a neuroma, but not every person says this happens.

Pain means different things to different people. What hurts one person is better tolerated by someone else. Gender, race and age influence pain differently. Pain is unpleasant and can reach a high level. A high pain score for neuroma would suggest an inability to concentrate, a state of anxiety, crying, intolerance to movement or pressure on the foot, or even an inability to wear shoes.

Discomfort is unpleasant but may be better tolerated. Because a neuroma affects a nerve, the sensation may be sharp or background dull; nerves provide a wide variety of sensations. Numbness is a useful indicator.

The common symptoms of neuroma are summarised below:

- Pain after walking/exercising
- Strange sensation under ball of foot and/or between toes
- Toes may swell or separate

- Electric shocks in toes
- Numbness
- Need to relieve pain by removing shoe

My story: After cycling, my foot experienced serious numbness between my third and fourth toes and under the foot. It was as if my foot had gone cold and I would have to wait for the circulation to come back... that was when I realised that I needed foot surgery.

Upon experiencing some type of symptom initially you might push the sole of your foot firmly with a finger, twiddle your toes and even squeeze and still not find pain.

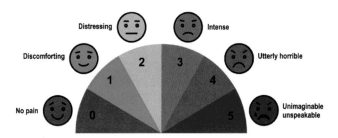

Figure 1.1
Visual Analogue Scale 0-5

If you cannot create the pain in your foot, what next?

This is the trial and error bit. Use different shoes and check when the symptoms occur. Keep a simple diary as part of your own analysis. If you want to use my journey diary (Section 6) you can, but it contains detailed narrative where simple notes might suffice. Your clinician may ask you similar questions to those listed below, so making notes from early on will improve your recall of detail. The diary may feature some of the points below. Record the level of pain using a scale 0-5 or 0–10, with 5/10 being the worst imaginable. The Visual Analogue Scale is used widely in healthcare to measure estimates of pain or discomfort. I have used a scale of 0–5 with smiley/sad faces in Figure 1.1. This gives an approximate idea of pain but not discomfort, which is subject to different influences such as movement rather than rest.

- When does it occur?
- Is the discomfort at the same time(s) of day?
- How long after waking does the pain take to emerge?
- Does it come and go?
- What makes it better (or worse)?
- Do you have one or more pair of shoes that make it worse?
- Is there an activity, social, athletic or professional action, that causes the problem?
- Could it be a change in your job?
- Does it happen when you drive?
- Is there a difference if you use an automatic gearbox over a manual gearbox (left foot mainly)?

My story: I coped for quite a while and I knew what it was, but it affected my cycling, especially after using a tighter pair of shoes. I had to use a bigger pair, which helped until riding a hill one day left me with a sensation like a local anaesthetic, causing numbness This included dull background pain as well.

Does the pain spread? Do you have any back problems? If the back has a known area of pain, then foot pain and numbness can be confusing because more than one nerve root might be affected. Nerves come out of the spinal cord like the branches of a tree. Some nerves, like the sciatic nerve, are long, thick and influence the foot. Nerve pain originating in another site, yet affecting the foot, is known as referred pain.

WHAT CAN I DO TO HELP MYSELF?

* Can you do more for yourself?
* Who do you see?

A neuroma is a damaged nerve affected by pressure, so anything you can do to alleviate that pressure will help. The good news is, if you can find the cause early enough the nerve will recover. Your aim is to do something before the nerve is irreversibly affected. Conservative treatment is more successful if used early.

Here are some options that can work early on.

MASSAGE
Especially in between the toes and up the foot (toward the ankle). It is best to rotate the fingers and use some creamy application or oil to assist your rubbing motion. Push down hard as well because the kneading effect encourages the blood supply, stimulating the healing response and desensitising the nerve (i.e., makes the nerve less sensitive).

ORTHOTIC INLAY

While the level of pain/discomfort is low, an arch support (inlay, insole, orthosis [the professional term]) can help. Avoid bulky inlays. The inlay shown in Figure 1.2 being raised does not lift the arch but helps alter the foot position and reduces the pressure under the ball of your foot. Three-quarter designs (shown) are better. Shoe fit can vary so your shoes must be deep enough. If pain or discomfort has reached the 4-5 mark, then inlays may not be tolerated. Figure 1.2 shows mid-price orthoses that can be bought via the internet or from reputable shops. Cheaper versions exist but designs that are too soft and flatten out may not work as well as firmer materials.

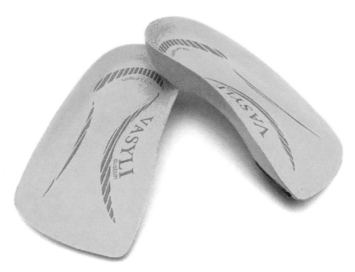

Figure 1.2
Orthotic Inlay bought from a pharmacy or internet
suppliers provides a cost effective method initially

Insoles can be helpful where a dome-shaped pad is fitted over the ball of the foot. It is possible to make something to stick to the foot or use a shop-bought inner sole made from a stiff leatherboard material. Chiropody felt can be cut to shape and placed on the inlay in true 'Blue Peter' style (see Figures 1.3 and Figure 1.4).

PRACTICAL PADDING FOR MORTON'S NEUROMA

The plantar metatarsal pad (PMP) will help (flexible) bent toes take pressure off the ball of the foot. This is not so successful for stiff bent toes.

HOW DOES THE PMP WORK?

The pressure under the metatarsal (see Figures 1.3 and Figure 1.4) is pushed upwards when the PMP is placed under the three central metatarsals. The metatarsal bones are pushed sideways, reducing impingement against the nerves. This is of particular value early in the diagnosis.

Note: Badly deformed, stiff toes require professional help.

Felt (white), usually 4–7mm thick, can be purchased from pharmacists or via the internet. The low-sensitive (hypoallergenic) adhesive backing is suitable for most skin types. Peel the back off after the pad has been cut to shape. The pad must align to the metatarsals exactly to work properly. Figure 1.3 indicates the shape and bevel (shaded edge marked by thick arrow) and Figure 1.4 provides an illustration of how to fit the pad to the location required. The dark shaded areas show how much the pad should be bevel trimmed to make it hug the foot better. The end towards the heel is made slightly shorter than the length of the metatarsal bones by 1.25cm, as shown using the the styloid process (marked) as a guide.

Finding the styloid process: It is easier to look at the outer side of the foot. Find where the foot starts to curve in. Moving back toward the ankle you will find the styloid process projects out at the end of the metatarsal.

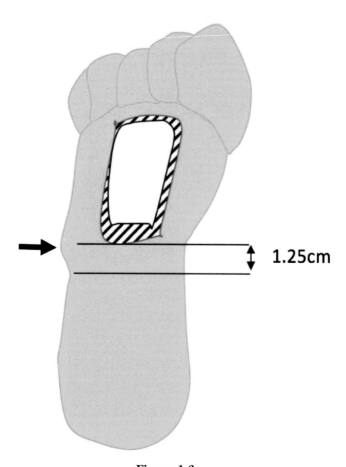

1.25cm

Figure 1.3
Placing the adhesive felt pad under the foot so that it
does not slip. Note the styloid process is a good point
seen at the location of the single head arrow. The
crease behind the arrow makes a reference point

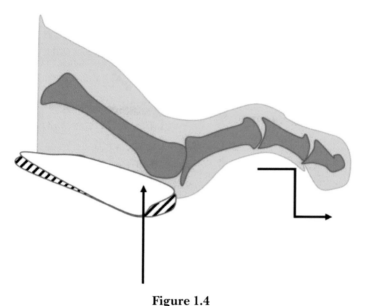

Figure 1.4
Shows a bevelled pad under the foot. Replace the pad
when it is no longer beneficial. Successful padding can
be upgraded to a quality orthotic inlay. The pad does not
need to be taped into place. Adhesive pads should not be
reused after soaking as movement can cause blistering.

Patients with poor circulation should seek professional advice first before using adhesive pads. The zig-zag
arrow in Figure 1.4 indicates that flexible (bent) toes
should lower after the pad has been fitted. In fixed toe
deformities they will not change position. Alternatives
exist and patients may prefer a ready made 'metatarsal
pad' pad; however there are a great many varieties on
the market. Most that I have viewed on the internet show
loose fitting inserts that may not help, although the older

leather metatarsal dome did work favourably. Thin pads collapse and will have little effect on toe position

MASSAGE WITH A SQUASH OR TENNIS BALL

This is best done after a warm bath or shower. Whilst sitting, press the ball up and down into the foot, and rotate the ball as shown by the arrows in Figure 1.5 to break up scar tissue formation and relieve spasm. Use your hand to push against the ball, or put the ball under the foot and use your downward weight. If you experience shooting pain, you know a nerve is trapped. If the nerve is too large, inflamed and tender you may have to stop. Some reflexologists can offer help by keeping management low key and hands on. The idea of the massage is to limit scar tissue formation.

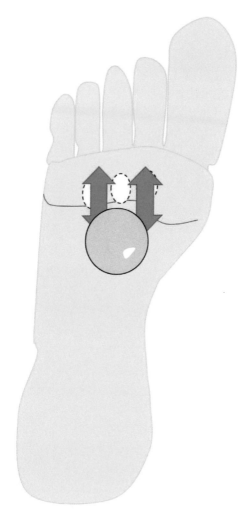

Figure 1.5
Using a ball for massaging in early
stages to reduce scar build up

FOOTWEAR

Try wearing shoes that have a slightly thicker sole than normal. If your foot changes size during the day, alter the fastening or swap between two different sized pairs of shoes. Avoid high heels as these cause nerve compression. Use your diary and act upon your findings to remove any factors that cause your foot pain.

Self-help does not seem to make a difference: what do I do next?
By now the nerve is thicker and may not recover. You will need medical guidance.

Six weeks is an ideal time to wait to see how your foot progresses with your own efforts to improve foot comfort. If you have constant or increasing symptoms seek help. Of course it may not be a neuroma so keep an open mind. If you have constant symptoms DO NOT wait. Try taking ibuprofen 400mg by mouth for 72 hours to see if there is any improvement, but <u>do not use this medication if you are allergic or have stomach problems</u>. If in doubt wait to see your GP before taking oral medicine.

If tablets such as ibuprofen (known as an anti-inflammatory) work, the condition should settle fast, suggesting that it is not a neuroma as anti-inflammatories do not cure neuromata. Rubbing an anti-inflammatory gel on the skin over the area is worth trying but don't be surprised if any benefits are short-lived, which is typical for this type of problem. These medications do not need a prescription. Do note that unbranded (generic) products are cheaper and just as effective.

WHO TO SEE?

Free: Your GP – your family physician knows a lot about many things but may not know about the foot in detail. He or she will know who to send you to but remember GPs will want to do all they can first to help you.

Paying: Can you go to someone else? Of course you can but then you will be outside the NHS system, which is free. If you are insured, you could go to a consultant who specialises in foot health, but ensure you have insurer approval first. Insurers no longer need a GP referral, but consultants prefer this method as it is important that good communication continues between GP and specialist.

You can select either a podiatric surgeon (Fellow of the College of Podiatry [Surgery]) or an orthopaedic surgeon (Fellow of the Royal College of Surgeons). Make sure the person you select specialises in feet. Orthopaedic surgeons may be members of the British Orthopaedic Foot and Ankle Surgery Society (BOFAS). If you are uncertain about who to see, discuss this with your GP who will almost certainly know the foot specialists in your area.

Podiatrists deal with the foot and can provide orthotic inlays and assist you with conservative care plans for your neuroma. Physiotherapists, chiropractors and osteopaths also provide orthotic inlays but may not specialise in this facet of care, and this could delay your treatment journey. I am of course biased as podiatrists are 100% dedicated to feet, take exams in medicine and anatomy and know about other parts of the body.

'I visited an exhibition and someone put me on a special pressure sensor and advised me to have a foot orthosis because this can help.'

Caution: use registered professionals[5] only

Is this a good idea?'

If this person is not a registered health professional, i.e., with the Health Care Professional Council (HCPC) or General Medical Council (GMC), then be cautious as you may have no comeback.

Health Care Professions Council registered (HCPC)	Podiatric surgeons, podiatrists, physiotherapists, radiographers, operating department practitioner
General Medical Council registered (GMC)	Medical (GP) doctors, orthopaedic surgeons, general surgeons, anaesthetists
General chiropractic Council & General Osteopathic Council registered (GCC & GOC)	Two separate professions; chiropractors and osteopaths

Table 1.1

Musculo-skeletal practitioners in the UK and their regulators[6]. <u>Note</u> nurses are registered by the Nurse & Midwifery Council (NMC) not by the HCPC or GMC

PRESSURE (FORCE) PLATES

Your patient journey may require diagnostic tests. Methods used to measure pressure or foot loads are enormously unpredictable depending on accuracy, cost, calibration and position of the equipment, and should be conducted by qualified people with clinical experience. The use of such a system looks impressive but correct interpretation is important. The safe choice? Go to your GP or direct to a foot care specialist.

What can you expect next?

If your symptoms interfere with your daily life you are now ready to do something. Do not pretend the pain will go. The earlier you act the greater the chances for resolution. However, if you cannot give much information or are vague, your consultation might be disappointing, or you simply walk away with painkillers. A consultation is made up of two parts: taking a history and examining the foot. Both have to be undertaken at the same time.

TIP – HELP YOUR DOCTOR

Use your notes from your diary. Patients who are organised are popular and allow the healthcare professional to focus in on their specific problem and make more efficient use of the consultation time.

How long has your condition been present? When does it happen? What makes it worse? Have you had treatment? Have you taken any medication? These are questions you should know the answers to.

Be aware of the timeline for a neuroma

MEDICAL HISTORY

As any medical disease affects your general health the progress of any foot condition must be considered within your medical history. Neuroma is a musculo-skeletal (MSK) condition. This means that it lies within the skeleton upon which bones move around joints, muscles lie in areas of the skeleton to move joints, and nerves and blood vessels supply muscles, joints and the skin. Your MSK condition is also important as it can provide a route whereby other conditions could mimic foot pain. The back is the big area for confusion, which I touched on in regard to nerve roots. This is why you need to consult someone with wide MSK experience (Table 1.1). Special areas for foot concern include diabetes, rheumatoid arthritis, ankylosing spondylitis, muscular and neurological diseases, some congenital conditions like club foot and spina bifida. Knowledge of a co-existing medical condition is important to planning treatment and providing quality advice.

THE EXAMINATION

This is broken down into:

Walking – a limp confirms that the body fails to move correctly and is likely to strain your musculo-skeletal frame. No one should limp without a reason.

Feeling and moving the foot – the area most common to Morton's neuroma is around toes 2–4. The bones and joints need to be examined and there will be some touch testing. I like to tap the main ankle nerve in case pain emerges further back in the foot or up the leg. This is part of the check for referred pain. The squeeze test comes with the Mulder click test (Section 2).

Seasoned professionals absorb information quickly and the examination process is learned over years of training in clinical practice. I have not listed every element the clinician needs to consider, but I do want to reassure you that professionals use a large amount of information to make the right choice. After 40 years I learn as much by talking and listening to my patients for golden nuggets of information that help me make the right therapeutic decision.

DIAGNOSIS

Do not be surprised if you are asked to consider some form of pain medication first. If you have used an anti-inflammatory like ibuprofen as suggested above, you should be ahead of the game. Tell your doctor you have tried this already, giving the dose, frequency and how long you have used it for. There is little point continuing if medication has failed already.

Treatment cannot start until a neuroma has been confirmed. This means a test. An X-ray might help rule

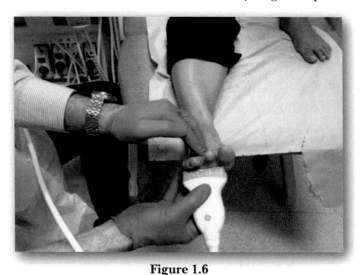

Figure 1.6
Ultrasound conducted using gel against skin provides a picture of the deep fat and increased fluid which may suggest a neuroma or bursa is present. The size of interruption can be measured. (Courtesy Holdcroft & Almallah, Walsall Healthcare NHS Trust. Poster presentation 2013)

out a secondary problem; for example, does your toe joint have some bone damage? An ultrasound does not use X-rays; a silent wave form bounces signals to reveal increased fluid content suggesting inflammation. The diagnostic version of ultrasound is helpful for nerves and bursae (fluid-filled sacs that reduce friction between tendons and bones); if the latter become inflamed it leads to a condition known as bursitis. It should not be confused with the treatment versions favoured by the physiotherapy profession.

OTHER METHODS OF INVESTIGATION

Occasionally clinicians prefer to use magnetic resonance imaging or MRI. We might call ultrasound and MRI, 'scans'. MRI is more complicated and uses electricity and magnets to alter the chemical structure (oxygen and hydrogen atoms) harmlessly. It also makes a lot of noise. Only the foot and lower leg go in a tunnel, not the whole body, so do not panic if you have claustrophobia.

X-rays and scans form the main tests.

Sometimes a dye might be used to enhance the picture. Imaging, as we call the above, will be carried out by the imaging department (radiology). Other professionals are qualified in the use of ultrasound but it is preferred to rely on the radiologist (medical doctor) for the interpretation, so you will end up with a clinical examination conclusion and a radiological examination conclusion. We aim to hit 95% accuracy with our tests.

SUMMARY

This section has considered the condition of neuroma, a painful foot condition affecting the nerves between bones called metatarsals. A nerve that is pinched causes a wide range of symptoms, including electric shocks called paraesthesiae. If the discomfort is constant you will need help. However, if the condition is recognised early, much can be done to remedy the discomfort and even reverse the condition. I have emphasised the following points:

- What to look for: pain specific to toes and ball of the foot, especially between toes 2-3 and 3-4, or splaying of toes
- The Visual Analogue Pain scale is helpful (Figure 1.1)
- Chief symptoms alleviated by removal of the shoe and a need to rub the foot
- A diary is useful and can help keep track of factors that make the foot worse. Try to eradicate things that cause problems.
- 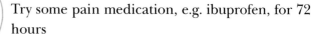 Try some pain medication, e.g. ibuprofen, for 72 hours

  (avoid on empty stomach or if you have gastro-intestinal problems or take other drugs such as blood thinners). Always read the information leaflet supplied.

- Change shoes, use thicker soles and alter activity that causes symptoms
- Buy a cheap inlay (insole) with slight inner raise
- Use a felt or shop-bought metatarsal pad to see if this helps toe alignment
- Seek professional advice direct from a podiatrist, foot orthopaedist or GP
- Consultation and diagnostic planning will end with a treatment plan

In the next section we need to discuss what a neuroma is and overcome confusion around diagnosis.

What exactly is a neuroma?

INTRODUCTION

THIS SECTION STANDS ALONE, so if you have skipped Section 1 that's fine as further points about treatment are covered later in Section 3. If you have reached a professional by this point an understanding of what a neuroma is will help when discussing treatment and increase your confidence when making decisions. If this section holds no interest, please move on to treatment in Section 3.

- Why are women more likely to experience a neuroma than men?
- Is it all to do with footwear?
- Are there any myths?

How does it feel?

By the time you have a diagnosis, months or even years may have passed before the damage reaches a critical point. You now have some idea of how it feels from Section

1: variable pain at one location between the second and third or third and fourth toes, under the foot, stinging at the end of toes, or electric shocks, a strange sensation bringing numbness that comes and goes. Spasm may come and go. A need to take the shoe off and rub the foot is a characteristic feature of neuroma. Disablement can be progressive.

My story: my neuroma probably started seven years earlier. The odd twinge made me suspect a problem but then it would go I ignored what was already set in motion...

KEY

MN: Morton's neuroma

    B: bursa

    Lig: metatarsal ligament

    Branch: where the nerves meet (dotted arrow)

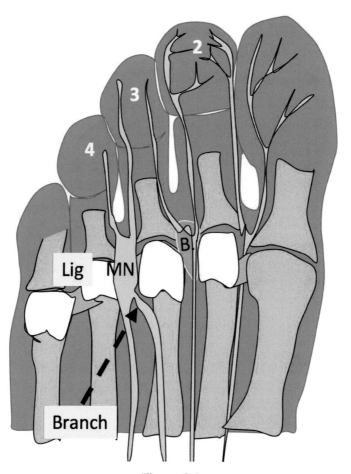

Figure 2.1
Nerve distribution to the second, third and fourth toes between the metatarsal heads (white)

The diagram in Figure 2.1 allows you to identify the two locations where pain arises: a Morton's[7] neuroma or a bursa (B). The foot has five long bones called metatarsals that are anchored from the mid-foot (not shown). At the end of each metatarsal a large surface area forms the weight- bearing ball of the foot. The toes are formed from three smaller bones in front of each metatarsal (phalanges – partially shown). These should be flexible and not stiff.

The nerves (yellow) actually start in the lower spine just above the pelvis but then run down the leg, around the ankle and into the foot. As the nerves near the ball of the foot, two nerves affecting the third and fourth toes become pinched at a common point where they join. This forms a junction box of sorts.

The diagram, while not strictly anatomically correct, emphasises the nerve branch. While only the main nerves supplying the second, third and fourth toes have been drawn, the fourth and fifth toes have a similar nerve distribution. The lack of detail is intended to avoid confusion and focuses on the three central toes (marked); second, third and fourth.

Figure 2.1 shows the small ligaments that prevent the bones from splaying, which can happen with age, pregnancy or weight gain. These are the intermetatarsal ligaments labelled Lig. It has been suggested that these ligaments can trap the nerve, causing the type of symptoms experienced by patients with neuromata. Keyhole surgery has been proposed to release this; it will be worthwhile coming back to this later, and is relevant to the next question.

Why is the nerve susceptible at this point?
The foot has two main nerve branches, one on the inside (medial) and the other on the outside (lateral) of the foot. Where the two branches join (see branch in Figure 2.1), the nerve is most susceptible to pressure. This occurs at the junction box mentioned previously.

Neuroma is a feature of the family of forefoot conditions called metatarsalgia, which comprises more than just Morton's. As seen in Figure 2.1, when the nerves reach the end of the toes they fan out like the branches of a stag deer's antlers. The pulp, or bulbous part has a greater nerve network than the top of the toe, which has a different nerve branch. Interference along any part of this nerve can cause symptoms reflected at the end of the toe. The pulp has a high fat density (yellow) and is supplied by pressure sensors and other refined nerve endings. This complements the body's radar system (Figure 2.2). Three types of sensory information are shown in the diagram. The schematic drawing of the end of a toe shows how the plantar (lower) nerve branch supplies most of the end of the toe, and is more sensitive to discomfort because of the extensive network of nerve endings. The specialised nerves provide additional information to the brain.

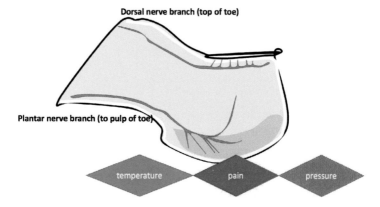

Figure 2.2
The plantar nerve branch

Why do I feel pain in the end of my toe and not near the nerve?
Conduction of nerve signals is interfered with where the medial and lateral branches join and radiate a signal toward the toe. However, we can record radiating discomfort shooting up toward the ankle or even leg as well. The objective of treatment is to take pressure away from the nerve, preventing it from becoming pinched before damage becomes permanent. If you use the plantar metatarsal pad described in Figure 1.4, this damage can be minimised. Likewise, an orthotic inlay can help achieve the same aim and was the reason my foot could be kept comfortable for so long.

I experience symptoms in my second/third toe. Is this the same as Morton's neuroma?
The simple answer is yes. Looking at diagram Figure 2.1 where a bursa [B] is represented, a sac of fluid fills the gap acting as a cushion between the second and third metatarsals. This condition, although similar, does not have the same nerve branch design, but if the bursa becomes inflamed, the nerve is compressed as in the third/fourth metatarsal space. Once the sac deflates, the pressure is relieved. Samples sent for microscopic analysis confirm 'bursa' as the diagnosis. This means sometimes the problem is nerve related and sometimes bursa related. Metatarsalgia pain can affect the second/third space as well as the third/fourth space but only the one located in the third/fourth space is

officially called Morton's. Symptoms can affect the end of any of these three central toes because of nerve signal interference.

What is the Mulder click test?

Once this test was considered to be the gold standard in diagnosing a neuroma, but now we combine it with other investigations and clinical history. In Mulder's test the metatarsals are squeezed to replicate shoe pressure. Enlarged nerves and bursae, shown in Figure 2.1, will pop between the metatarsals and ligaments, often making shoes uncomfortable. The test is positive for both bursae(plural) and neuromata.

Is a neuroma a tumour?

A neuroma has features of a normal nerve but abnormal inflammation and scar tissue exist. A tumour arises from abnormal cells and can be harmless (benign) or harmful (malignant). Like the bricks of a house, cells make up our bodily structure and give us shape and support. Cells have a centre called a nucleus, a watery medium inside and a wall outside called a membrane. The inside nucleus can be faulty leading to abnormal development. A neuroma does not have the same features as a tumour; the word tumour is derived from the ancient Greek word for 'swelling'.

Can neuromas (neuromata) become malignant?

I have seen plenty of neuroma reports and in 30 years of operating have never seen a case of malignancy[8] where the initial diagnosis was a neuroma. However, we have to be open minded. As far as I am aware conscientious surgeons send all tissue samples off just in case there is cause for concern, but the risk is negligible. The other reason to investigate the piece of tissue is to define our own diagnosis, which means the course of care and outcome should be predictable.

If it is not a neuroma what can it be?

The most common condition to mimic neuroma is synovitis, as shown in Figure 2.3. The space between the bones becomes pressed by swelling inside the joint. This condition is called synovitis, or inflammation of the lining of the joint where joint lubrication is produced.

When this is not case we have to consider other courses that may involve a nerve in some way: diabetes, vitamin B12 deficiency, other blood conditions, nerve problems associated with the back or trapped nerves around the ankle. These conditions are outside the remit of this book. Even the most experienced foot specialists can be baffled.

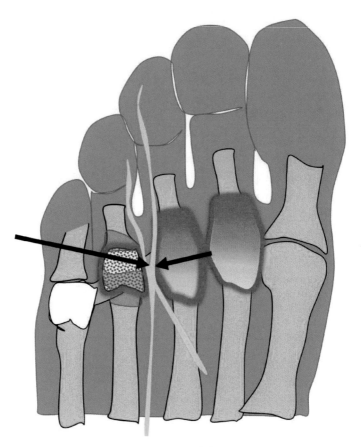

Figure 2.3
Swelling of the joint capsule (red). The
diagram is again drawn to show the main nerve
only affected by compression of fluid

Why are women more susceptible to Morton's neuroma or neuroma affecting the second/third toes?

For the most part footwear design is blamed for pain. Fashionable' shoes in particular have two design features that conflict with the needs of the foot's internal bone –joint structure: tight toe boxes in heels.

Shoemakers expect the front of the foot (the toebox) to be sufficiently tight so as not to loosen. Some feet, though not all, will push against the nerves at 2-3 or 3-4 (see Figure 2.4), creating those changes. Ligaments that might prevent splaying of bones cannot stop the same bones pushing together.

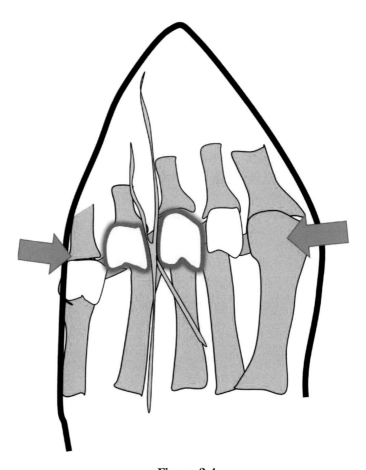

Figure 2.4
The effect of shoe compression on the nerve becomes more notable with bunion deformities and tight toe box designs

Heels

As heel height increases, let's say for the sake of argument over 3.75cms, the three central metatarsal bones 2-3-4 (the ball) are exposed to significant pressure so that the nerves are nipped between bones and joints. Shoe compression is worse with thin soles.

Bunion

The presence of a bunion deformity widens the foot and makes it take up more room in the shoe. It is not uncommon to find women with a bunion deformity (hallux valgus) that has to be accommodated in a standard shoe. A neuroma between both the second-third and third-fourth toes can already be present, or can be further exacerbated by the overall tight compaction. What might have appeared as one condition now appears as two or more.

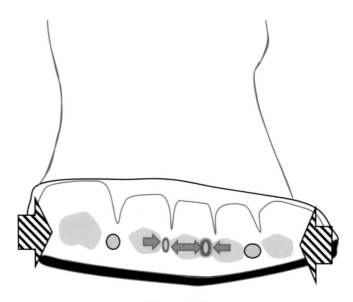

Figure 2.5
The effect of shoe compression seen from
the toe end with shoe superimposed

Why do men suffer if they don't wear tight shoes?

Injury, twisting the foot and hurting the forefoot can set up symptoms in the absence of footwear- created problems, but they are not recognised in traditional literature reports. Men can still use tight shoes, not realising a problem exists; one pair might do more damage than expected. When Peter (not his real name) asked me to help him, his foot was incredibly painful. He had gone beyond the point of no return and was not only frustrated, but had to persuade his GP to refer him.

Orthoses and conservative care were too late to help Peter as his condition was too advanced. The interesting thing was Peter worked in surgery with me so I was able to follow his care. Peter was just six months ahead of me (Section 6).

Muscle spasms: The small bones and joints of the front of the foot have tiny muscles that attach to each side of the toe to supplement other muscles. Strap-like muscles called interossei can go into spasm causing pain for short periods.

My story: I would not have believed that spasm could affect the nerve but have been converted realising to me that this is what happened to me. I had a bout a spasm, often at night in bed. I suggest that sufficient spasm (tightening) of the fibres within the muscle can impact on the nerves 2-3 and 3-4, influencing the nerve overtime.

FOOT TYPES

It has long been proposed that certain foot types can cause or influence a neuroma. A bunion overcrowds the front of the foot contributing to foot pain. Toe deformities (e.g., hammer toes) push the metatarsals down, making the ball more prominent.

First metatarsal

My radiologist (X-ray doctor) always likes to point out metatarsals that are too close together and believes this creates a likely problem for neuromata. When asked to give a lecture abroad in November 2016, I looked at 'Myths, Facts and Fables' as a subject matter and found several articles on the length of metatarsals. In fact, another Morton (Dudley) suggested in 1927 that there was a difference between the *Greek* foot and the *Egyptian* foot. The idea was determined by the first metatarsal having a different length (see Figure 2.6). He classified the two feet by the known length of the first and second metatarsals. In the figure the sketch shows the five metatarsals and an X-ray is presented for comparison. The first metatarsals are distinctly shorter than the second metatarsals. Not believing the myth, I explored past patients and recalled their X-rays to find there was some truth to this length of bones theory: if you have a short first metatarsal and a relatively long second metatarsal, then a neuroma may well arise.

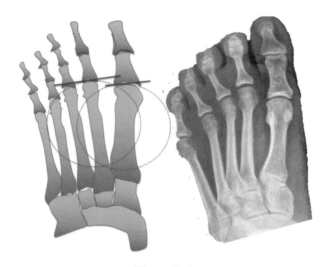

Figure 2.6
The short first metatarsal shape: Greek foot
Illustration of an actual x-ray. Red lines show length
difference between the first and second metatarsals.

THE FOOT SHAPE

Other types of feet include flat feet, but there is another foot condition called pes cavus that is represented by a high arch. The flat foot can provoke neuroma symptoms but alone this is not necessarily a common feature. Toe deformities and wide feet are key to the problem with a bunion deformity. High arch feet are different as severe forms of stiff toe deformity arise, causing pronounced pressure under the ball of the foot. Unless you have the misfortune to have a severe foot deformity affecting the toes, the chances are that you will not suffer from neuromata any more than anyone else no matter what arch shape you have.

My toes are splayed, does this mean anything?

In Section 1 I touched on splayed toes. Some patients have natural spaces between their toes, but more often splaying means the metatarsal ligaments are stretched, or a muscle is poor at stabilising the toe, or the toe has some local swelling so that an enlarged bursa [B] (Figure 2.1) can push the toes apart. Measurement of the neuroma after an ultrasound can show progress or deterioration when a review is considered. Expect to have an ultrasound diagnostic test repeated before surgery unless it is patently obvious in the first place.

Bunion (a co-existing problem)

Although I have already alluded to the bunion, room for greater detail is unavailable in a book on neuroma as this subject would be too extensive. However, a question about treatment of the bunion will crop up during your examination for neuroma and may even be the reason for your consultation. Little is written about the incidence of bunion deformity with pain under the ball of the foot. Foot surgeons may undertake surgery for both conditions together, or treat separately. The decision is as always based on symptoms and the evidence available at the time. The facts that do seem to ring true are as follows:

* A broad foot is susceptible to a neuroma in spaces 2-3, 3-4

- Bunion deformities (hallux valgus) disturb toe alignment, causing pain under the ball of the foot
- Pain after bunion surgery may develop under the ball (metatarsals) and appears as a complication. Recovery from surgery may have exacerbated an existing neuroma problem.
- If the neuroma was pre-existing before bunion surgery the choice to treat should be discussed with your foot specialist

PATIENT EXPERIENCES

Some patients put off having treatment. I think they fear the worst and certainly fear surgery. Fear can interfere with making a timely decision. Naturally there are bad stories that play on fear. Exposure to a bad story is frightening and is why dedicated specialists are generally better at managing a neuroma. They have depth of knowledge through experience and are likely to have more compassion and motivation. Having surgery myself was an eye opener and improved my clinical judgement. Common questions could help reassure patients when progress is slow. Wendy returned to see me two years after she first complained of pain and had never been keen for an operation. Her comment when the pain became so bad:

'I think you are right, Mr Tollafield -this is not going to get better.'

If you are going to delay treatment you need to know what to expect and know the limitations of conservative treatment (Section 3).

A CLOSER LOOK AT NERVES

What happens to a nerve to make it so painful?

It may help to see what the real nerve looks like and then we can look at a schematic drawing to pick up the main features. Nerves are small structures and there is little space between toes and joints to accommodate any increase in size. Figure 2.7 is a real picture of a neuroma removed from one of my patients. The surgical clips are holding the two branches that supply the second-third toes. The main body has a heavy deposit of fat to insulate the nerves from damage during walking. As it is essentially a digital nerve, the term digital neuritis or even inter-digital neuritis has being used. The end that is still attached can have a long tail that runs between the metatarsals. The nerve thickens and becomes less effective at conducting.

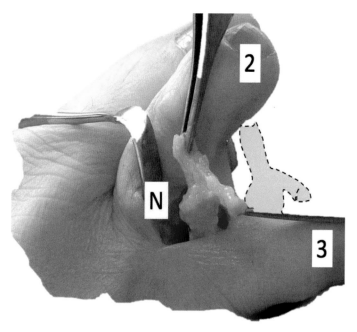

Figure 2.7
Nerve removed between the second and third toes. The
offset yellow diagrammatic impression provides a general
outline of the branches to the toes.
N - NERVE

What does the (inter)digital nerve do?

A nerve conducts a signal in a similar way to a wire conducting electricity. Both use electrical impulses that relay messages quickly. Voluntary nerves influence movement around a joint, while involuntary nerves perform functions such as influencing the diameter of a blood vessel in response to temperature fluctuations. The digital nerve picks up information using specific endings like a radar. There are a number of different nerves specialising in information about touch (pressure), temperature (hot and cold), vibration and pain (Figure 2.2). It seems logical that if this nerve is removed then all this sensory information will disappear, but it is important to grasp that sensations may be altered depending upon which areas are affected.

Are nerves important

Nerves provide information as suggested above. A small loss of information is not critical, but may be irritating as sensation is depleted. For prospective surgery nerve sensation loss will be discussed in later chapters.

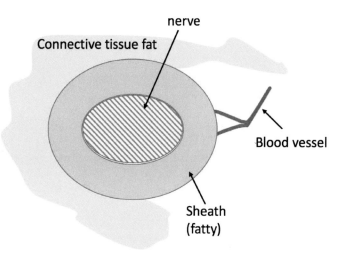

Figure 2.8
Normal nerve in cross-section (schematic impression)

Can we sacrifice sensations?

The answer is yes; we can sacrifice one for the other. Loss of sensation over small areas is well tolerated and common following surgery where skin is cut. Some sensation may return after about nine months. Loss of power to move muscles should not occur. A 'spacetomy' is a colloquial term to describe the procedure where all the muscles and nerves are removed between metatarsals. This was a hammer-to-crack-a-nut analogy and imprecise. There is no need to move muscle bulk even if these muscles are small. There are some basics we need to be aware of. In the next diagram (Figure 2.8) a loose interpretation of the nerve is shown, with it surrounded by a fatty sheath with little gaps at intervals (not shown) called nodes. This fatty covering allows messages

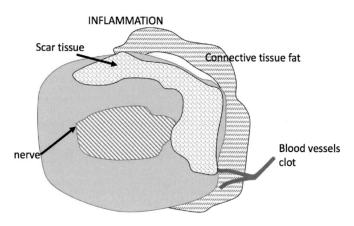

Figure 2.9
Abnormal nerve in cross-section (schematic impression)

to travel quickly, jumping across the gaps. If the sheath is damaged messages fail to travel normally but can be amplified unhelpfully.

SYMPTOMS OF NEUROMA

One sign of abnormal nerve travel is an electrical sensation called a paraesthesiae. Sudden shock arises when you catch the foot awkwardly or walk on uneven 'bobbly' surfaces. Not only does the impulse from the nerve signal seems harsh but it can travel into the toe or back up the foot I have known patients find the sensation runs up the leg.

How do we know about the nerves altering?

Nerve studies are not new, and they can be tested for the speed that impulses travel. This is not important for small nerves like a digital neuroma. We rely on our colleagues who study pieces of tissue under a microscope after removal. The size the nerve grows to is affected by scar tissue[9]. Blood flow becomes blocked in the tiny vessels (Figure 2.9). This leads to repair and formation of scar tissue. The downward spiral is now set in motion as the nerve sheath is rendered inefficient and signals are altered unhelpfully. The neuroma is now just a rather useless nerve causing pain.

Summary

Section 2 has provided information about the cause of nerve deterioration. This will help you understand treatment better.

- Gender differences: women are 4-6 times more likely to suffer than men
- Shoes contribute unhelpfully if they are too tight, the heel is too high or the sole too thin
- Neuromata are common in patients affected by bunion deformity due to pressure and lack of space in tighter shoes
- Neuroma can be caused by injury. Scar tissue formation commonly arises. Muscle spasm can compress the nerve.
- Foot shape- metatatarsal bone length, bunions and high arch feet with rigid toe deformities can pinch nerves
- Nerves provide sensory information from the pulp of the toe about pressure, temperature and vibration, acting as a radar for the brain
- Loss of sensation is not as important as disabling pain
- Nerve damage – the nerve enlarges, loses its blood supply, scars and fails to work normally
- Neuroma is sometimes called digital neuritis or metatarsalgia

- Treatment can reduce pressure, improve poor toe positioning and reduce compression of nerves. Surgery is not always necessary.
- Deformities such as broad forefeet and bunions may have to be treated in order for the neuroma to be dealt with

The next section deals with working on a treatment plan.

What treatment can I expect?

INTRODUCTION

IF YOUR SYMPTOMS HAVE CREATED discomfort and disability, treatment is inevitable and invasive procedures might be the preferred route. Conservative management should be considered within the diagnostic process, and needs to be discussed before opting for any surgery.

Risks from invasive treatment are dealt with in Section 4 so you can jump to the next part if surgery has already been decided and you are at the final consent stage.

DISABILITY

Perhaps we all think of wheelchairs and crutches when thinking of disability. Disability is a state where our performance slows down and simple activities are difficult to achieve. Disablement from a neuroma can vary. Pain and discomfort may only be an occasional feature. Later the frequency of symptoms affects regular activities such as shopping, walking and climbing stairs. Some of my patients have been drawn to tears with discomfort and frustration by what appeared as a simple condition. It is important to consider how the condition affects you, and how to exorcise the problem.

Treat early – avoid surgery. Ignore it – risk deterioration!

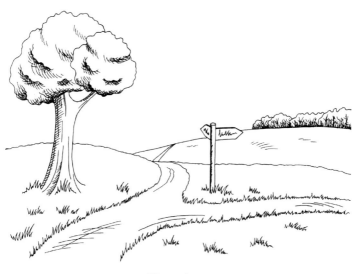

The pathway

Pathway

What we now call a pathway is also called the care plan, and more recently because of more patient focus, the patient journey.

Never jump into surgery without:

a) understanding clearly what it is you are suffering from

b) agreeing in your heart to the process of treatment prescribed

I personally feel patients should go away to consider the ramifications of what has been said during the consultation before saying 'Yes'. Better still, bring someone with you – a friend or family member – as it is easy to miss what has been said, especially if it is not what you want to hear.

Curiously this is where some patients misunderstand what is truly required, which can lead to a deterioration in their relationship with the specialist down the line. Can I avoid surgery?

Yes, you can always avoid surgery where a condition is not life threatening. The choice is yours and no one else's. Patient's must not be cajoled into surgery, although it is clear that foot surgeons sometimes hint that there is no alternative. I am always keen patients should see a podiatrist before coming to me as my speciality is surgical management. Healthcare is now too complex to suggest everything is known. From a clinician's point of view we tend to stick with what works most of the time.

My story: Did I want surgery on my foot? Absolutely not. I was not frightened but I knew all the consequences ahead, and also being busy I could not afford the time away from work. Like most, I had pressures and deadlines to meet.

I will pick up decision making again in another section, but we need to consider the three phases of a management pathway:

* Self-help (I have covered self-care in Section 1)
* Conservative active care
* Invasive management

SELF-HELP

The patient is directly involved with managing their own care. We learned that massage can help inflammation and scar tissue. Orthotic inlays are recommended where the pain scale, called a visual analogue scale, is low around 1 or symptoms infrequent. I suggested that a diary was used to check the influence of activity, shoes and any other factors influencing your condition. A reflexologist[10] was suggested as an alternative therapy; a formal body for the practice exists, the British Reflexology Association - http://www.britreflex.co.uk

Look to your occupation or social activities and remove any factor that makes your symptoms worse. Self care, however, has limited effects when the neuroma (what we call a lesion) has progressed to emit pain on a regular basis.

INVESTIGATIONS AND CONSULTATION

If you have not had the benefit of reading this book before your clinical discussions then fact sheets will have been provided, or you may have done some online research for yourself. X-rays do not show soft tissue such as a neuroma but they can exclude other problems, including healed hairline fractures. An MRI may have been used, sometimes with a dye to make the lesion clearer.

My story: As a clinician I have used MRI and found no neuroma, then during surgery discovered a large neuroma. This test is a false negative in this case. Be aware some investigations are not 100% reliable. Your clinician/specialist has to make decisions just as I did. Should I operate or not? Because of the reliability issue, I find ultrasound more helpful and work with an experienced radiologist to read my scans. Again ultrasound is not perfect but it is reasonably specific for this type of lesion and sensitive to changes associated with inflammation and fluid build up. Differentiating between a bursa and a neuroma is not always possible but treatment is the same.

CONSERVATIVE ACTIVE CARE
INJECTIONS
Oh, I am not good with needles the patient tells me for the nth time.

I say, 'I know, it is normal to not like needles – who does?!

I try to reassure patients with practical responses, such as:

* This could cure you
* It takes moments to do
* I have done hundreds
* I have had an injection myself
* The needle I use is similar to the diameter of an acupuncture[11] needle
* I use an anaesthetic so you won't feel the substance going in

Out of these six statements, one is a fib. It is the last statement, but the fib is only perception of the truth. I use an anaesthetic and the needle pierces the skin as if it is going into butter and often is not noticed as it is so fine. I've done this to myself so I know what I am talking about.

As I inject the anaesthetic the local nerves register the pressure of the fluid as swelling increases with the volume injected. If there is any inflammation present, the local anaesthetic will sting. This is because the anaesthetic is slightly acidic to preserve the drug. The stinging sensation lasts for less than 30 seconds. Once done, the actual treatment, a steroid, is not noticed. The needle is placed around the nerve, not into the nerve.

WORRIES ABOUT STEROID
'*Steroids aren't good for you, are they?*'
I reply this is not that kind of steroid. You will not put on weight even though small amounts go into the bloodstream.

'*Yes, but they only work for a short period?*'
This is not strictly true but it can be. Let me explain. The injection of steroids will set about reducing both inflammation and swelling, but will also reduce the scar tissue around the nerve, allowing some recovery. I set up a study of 60 patients in 1988 and found that 38% benefitted beyond six months with a steroid. Those who didn't were provided with surgery.

'*I'm going abroad and the injection did help so please can I have another one to tide me over?*'
While the ethics behind this judgement might be queried, I am on the patient's side as another won't hurt, but it might not last long. I might also inject the joint to rule out inflammation causing pressure (Figure 2.2).

'Can I be worse off after an injection?'

Actually yes, you can, although it is unusual. Injections fail for several reasons. The most common reason is that the nerve swelling and damage will not resolve with an injection, and success may last for only a few days or weeks. That is actually helpful for the foot surgeon as we know we should not use more steroid. Injection into the nerve can cause pain for a while, although this is rare. A flare up creates a local inflammatory reaction where the body fights the drug and goes ballistic. This sort of pain can arise in 3–4% of patients, but more so with joint injections than with those for neuroma. Discomfort settles with local ice, rest and taking suitable pain medication (analgesics) within 72 hours.

'Could I get an infection?'

As needles are sterile infection is rare, as is chorioretinopathy affecting the eye following local administration of corticosteroids via intra-articular (joints) or topically (skin).

'What could arise if I have an infection?'

You may need time off work. Treatment with incorrect antibiotics could cause super- or supra-infections needing hospitalisation. While the risk of infection is low from a steroid injection, the impact is moderate if it is treated quickly.

During surgery some steroids create harmless deposits, and generally do not cause tissue damage.

'Do steroids work straight away?'

Steroids may take up to six weeks to work. I am emphasising this as it is not uncommon for patients to think it is a waste of time. It is not. I found my own injection was of immediate help because the local anaesthetic dulled the pain initially. It had an effective life span of two days. It was then that I knew surgery was the only outcome for me. I call this a positive diagnostic outcome. Patients rarely refuse an injection. It is quick to deliver and you can walk away – although a modicum of rest on the day is best. The injection is both therapeutic (treats) and diagnostic, i.e, it benefits the patient by showing how significant the nerve damage is.

WHAT OTHER CONSERVATIVE TREATMENTS EXIST?

Therapeutic ultrasound can reduce fluid and inflammation in the metatarsal interspace, but it is not regarded as a main stay treatment. Repeat treatment is necessary.

Reflexology and acupuncture[11] may have a part to play. I have seen reflexology work for one patient in the past, which is hardly an illuminating recommendation but she just did not want traditional treatment. Treatments are repeated.

Homeopathic drugs and similar. This is not within my own expertise and it is very much open to debate as to how effective such applications are beyond any placebo effect. A qualified homeopathic doctor[12] might be worth consulting if steroids and surgery causes anxiety. This form of management may be useful as an alternative to traditional analgesics/anti-inflammatories but is unlikely to do much for an established neuroma.

Injections with alcohol or sclerosing agents have been popularised in the USA. Both work by effectively damaging the nerve, while steroids help the nerve recover without damage. Such procedures do not have universal acceptance in the UK, but that does not mean that such treatments cannot be offered where the clinician has prior experience and is within his or her scope of care. In the USA many non-surgical procedures were developed historically because podiatrists were not able to perform surgery. It is therefore not unreasonable to suggest that such a trend may follow in the UK where similar treatments appear favourable. As with cryosurgery and radio-frequency ablation (see below), while low risks have been reported, the injections maybe conducted blind unless ultrasound is used.

INVASIVE PROCEDURES

The effectiveness of any procedure can only be determined by its frequency and popularity being reported in scientific journals, backed by acceptable use in regular healthcare, be it NHS, private/independent sector, and endorsed by Colleges and professional bodies where procedures are governed by ethical approval from internal and external committees, such as England's National Institute for Health and Care Excellence (NICE, nice.org.uk).

CRYOSURGERY

Used with a local anaesthetic, a ball of ice forms at the probe end, damaging the nerve and creating an inflammatory response. This is not something I do myself due to personal beliefs about blindly damaging tissue, but it is picking up interest in the UK. The procedure is popular in the USA, but UK-based websites containing further information can be found.

One site reported low complications and risks, but mentions abscess formation, mild infection, scarring, prolonged soreness and numbness. In reality these problems are universal to any invasive procedure, including surgery. Cryotherapy also has a shorter recovery period (so stated on one UK website) and does not completely destroy the nerve, and therefore does not usually result in permanent numbness of the foot or toes. I cannot comment on the value of cryosurgery as research studies are subject to further evaluation by NICE.

RADIOFREQUENCY ABLATION (RFA)

A little more information is available on RFA as a key-hole method, where a small hole is made through the skin for painful interdigital (Morton's) neuroma, which is usually done as an outpatient procedure under local anaesthesia. Using ultrasound, an RFA probe attached to a generator is inserted into the web space between the toes and into the area of the neuroma. Controlled pulses of radiofrequency energy are delivered, which cause heat destruction of the nerve. After the procedure a steroid injection is usually given to reduce pain and inflammation. Patients are discharged as soon as comfortable and advised to limit their walking for one or two days. Any pain is managed with analgesics. The procedure can be repeated if necessary after a few weeks.

When NICE considered RFA, it decided that 'there was not much good evidence about how well this procedure works'. The five studies that NICE looked at involved a total of 182 patients. Generally, most patients reported the following benefits up to 6-10 months after the procedure:

* Of 37 patients, most (84%) said that they would have the procedure again

- In one patient, symptoms came back nine months after treatment, but were successfully treated
- About 30% of patients in a study of 38 patients had no benefit and went on to have surgery to remove the nerve

The RFA studies showed that the risks of this treatment for Morton's neuroma included:

* infection
* nerve irritation
* blood-filled swelling
* burns caused by incorrect positioning of the probe
* NICE was also told about some other possible risks, including bruising, scarring around the nerve and destruction of bone tissue.

While these two newer invasive procedures offer faster recovery and can be done under local anaesthetic on a day-patient basis, so can surgery. I elected to have my surgery under general anaesthetic and went home later that morning, but the surgical operation known as a neurectomy can be performed under local anaesthetic. Read more about data[13] collection.

CUTTING THE INTERMETATARSAL LIGAMENT

Where the ligament between the metatarsal heads (Figure 3.1) impinges on the nerve, tension can be released via a small incision (keyhole). Again this approach promises quick recovery. I cannot claim experience here, neither do I know people who perform this, despite its attraction. Performing surgery blind without ultrasound or X-rays (fluoroscopy) is less popular. There are blood supply and post-surgery scar tissue problems to consider.

Ligament release will work better in the earlier stages of the condition. There are other invasive procedures where the ligament is separated so in reality this procedure is used in the traditional neurectomy described next.

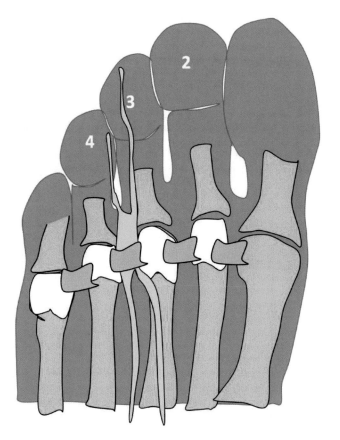

Figure 3.1
Intermetatarsal (bones) with ligaments
acting as struts to stop splaying

NEURECTOMY

The surgical procedure where the nerve is removed is called a neurectomy. Access can be from the top, inside the web of the toes, just under the toes or on the sole of the foot (Figure 3.2). The access method comes down to surgeon preference. This procedure has been carried out probably since 1893 and is well documented in the medical literature. Be prepared to have one foot operated on at a time. Your surgeon will discuss what is best.

Can I have both feet operated on at the same time?
Mobility after having surgery on both feet can make recovery challenging. Additionally, if you carry a little more weight, relying on crutches can be exhausting.

Can I have two neuromata taken out on the same foot?
It is possible to remove two neuromata at the same time, but the risk from healing problems increase when operated from the top of the foot as the blood supply to the middle toe can shut down. The risks increase with age and some medical diseases; we call this 'vascular embarrassment'. The decision to operate on two spaces at once is therefore not only based on an assessment of the risks, but is also down to surgeon preference.

The incision can be made over the third toe to gain access (point A in Figure 3.2), but any scarring can affect the joint and make the third toe joint stiff. An approach that tackles the problem of two spaces involves going in from the sole; we call this the sulcus of the toes. Incision F might provide better and safer access than one from the top. This cannot be done by keyhole surgery unless ultrasound is used. The reliability of this procedure has not yet been published to my knowledge. Incision line F may be modified and can join with either D or E to offer larger exposure. This forms an upside down 'U' shape.

Should I select my own operation site?

This should be considered along with the surgeon's advice as there may be practical reasons to select one incision site over another. There is no right or wrong way but there are reasons to help your understanding. Table 7.2 may be helpful in summarising the practicalities.

Incisions under the sole, at points D, E or F, may provide clearer visibility where parts of the nerve can be missed. Because ultrasound is used more frequently before surgery, the position of the nerve can be better planned. If the nerve sits under the metatarsal head, then an incision through the sole may be better. If the neuroma sits between the metatarsals, a top of foot incision (A–C) may be better for adequate access to the nerve.

The ligament (called the deep transverse ligament) sits over the nerve. If we operate from the top, the ligament must be cut to reach the nerve. When the sole is selected as the line of incision, the ligament can remain untouched.

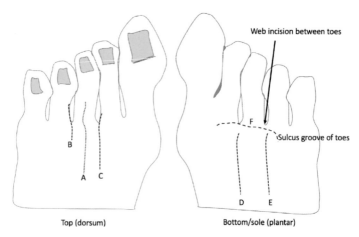

Figure 3.2
Common incision lines for neuroma surgery

My story: Taking another viewpoint, and one I considered important in making my decision, an incision on top of the foot may heal faster by a week. The risk from 'seed corn' formation is ever present with incisions under the sole. Refer to Section 5, where I discuss approaching from the sole in more detail.

THE SCAR ON THE FOOT

'It doesn't matter, it is only my foot and no-one will see it!'

An often misleading quoted line from patients. Scars are personal no matter where sited and can be painful, more so if a nerve is trapped within the scar formation. We don't know why but some scars, although fine in appearance to touch, can be sensitive; this is known as hypersensitivity.

Our aim

The scar should be neat, not ugly or raised, and it should be flat. The skin should not sparkle with hypersensitivity after lightly touching with finger pressure.

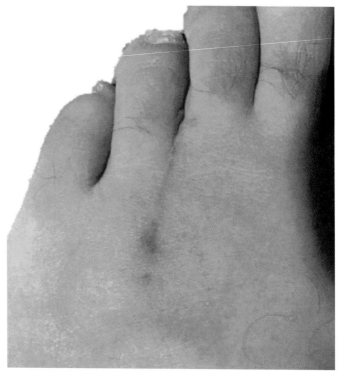

Figure 3.3
My foot at six months, all healed with skin blemish but the scar line is flat

The colour may be slightly different to the adjacent skin, but blend after 6–24 months. Scars can be difficult to predict as skin types come in different shades of quality and heal differently.

Why do 'blobs', as I call them, happen? The stitch (suture) absorbs and creates defence cell activity (white blood cells). Inflammation, if prolonged, may prevent the wound from healing.

My story: I heal pretty well but have a 'blob' at the end of my wound where the skin is discoloured, as shown in Figure 3.3. I had no infection but that bit of the scar took six weeks to settle. The delay surprised me but was exactly what I have found in operating on my own patients occasionally. The wound in my case is neat and will fade but I will always have a telltale sign. More about scars later when we discuss recovery.

TYPE OF ANAESTHETIC
LOCAL ANAESTHETIC (AS AT THE DENTIST)

No special theatre is required for admission into hospital for a local anaesthetic (LA) procedure. Many units exist as day care units in community centres. The foot is numbed up first by injecting nerves around the ankle. There maybe some discomfort from the initial injection but this soon settles and numbness follows up to an hour later. The only sensations are touch and pressure, and these are often vague but may lead to some patients requiring reassurance that they will not feel any pain. Many patients like this method as they stay awake, do not feel drowsy and there is minimal risk of nausea etc. There is no need to starve before this surgery, but a heavy meal beforehand is not recommended.

LOCALS ANAESTHETIC ASSISTED WITH SEDATION (THE HALF-WAY HOUSE)

The procedure is the same as above for LA but a plastic tube, called a cannula, is inserted into a vein and relaxing medication injected. Patients remain in control where confirmation is required but feel calm and probably sleepy. The medication may take a few hours to wear off. The benefits of this method are a low chance of being sick, you remember very little and if you are anxious this soon goes away. At no time do you need anything inserted into the throat, though an oxygen mask will be kept on throughout. Sedation has to be carried out in a registered centre as controlled drugs are used and licensed against abuse. Hospital day admission is usual and you will need to starve; see below. You will need someone to take you home afterwards as you may feel a little woozy.

General anaesthetic

All general anaesthetics in the UK are performed in a registered hospital with a medically qualified anaesthetist. They will take a medical history before surgery. The doctor will explain the process and make sure you are fit and have not eaten for 6–8 hours beforehand. This ensures there is no chance of food vomit entering the lungs. We like to have patients drink water up to two hours before surgery to keep them hydrated and minimise headaches. All anaesthetics are safe today, especially where patients are fit. There is a lower chance of sickness with modern anaesthetics. The RCoA's website[14] has a complete list of the risks and side effects of anaesthesia.

Neurectomy procedures take 15–25 minutes in experienced hands, so 30–40 minutes is the length of time you will probably be asleep for.

Do I have a choice of anaesthetic?

Yes, to some extent. In a day unit local anaesthetic may be the only option. If you are anxious, consider sedation as this is very effective. Some surgeons prefer general anaesthetic and feel less comfortable using LA.

Older patients with complex medical history, or breathing problems such as severe asthma, will do better with LA and light sedation. General anaesthetic can take some patients longer to recover from and smokers often require a higher dose of anaesthetic.

SUMMARY

This section has considered a range of treatments, divided into self care, conservative active care by a professional and invasive care. The use of steroids is an important part of management. There are some warnings, listed below.

MORE INFORMATION ABOUT STEROIDS

- Steroid injections carry fear but offer a valuable method to recover nerves
- Repeat injections do not work as well as the first injection
- Injecting into another area at the same time is perfectly fine
- Large amounts of steroid when repeated can actually do harm, thinning the fat tissue and causing dimpling or making the skin thin and discoloured
- Infection is rare and likely to be pre-existing

Essential points relating to other treatments

- The decision for treatment rests with the patient
- Pain greater on a visual analogue scale of 2/5 or 4/10 is indicative that the problem is deteriorating
- Information should help to inform and is part of the consent process

- Orthotic inlay trials are important but fail to work where the nerve is irreparably damaged
- Reflexology, therapeutic ultrasound, acupuncture, homeopathic therapy and injections with alcohol and sclerosing agents can be considered but are not all widely available in the UK or proven to be of any real benefit
- Keyhole (closed) procedures such as cryosurgery and radiofrequency ablation have value but long-term information is currently not available. Both procedures are not without risk.
- Ligament release may be helpful, dependent on how far the nerve has deteriorated
- Surgery by an invasive method has existed since the 19th century, forming an open procedure and healing in 2–6 weeks.
- Access to the foot is from the sole or top of the foot
- Surgery by experienced foot surgeons has a high success rate
- Anaesthetic choices are available to patients; each has different advantages and all are carried out with day surgery in mind
- Operating with single incisions on one foot at a time lowers the risk from surgery
- Wounds may take over 12 months to settle completely and can remain discoloured.

In the next section consent for and risks of neurectomy surgery are considered.

Neurectomy. Consent and risks. Knowing what to expect

INTRODUCTION

CONSENT IS A PROCESS THAT allows you to make a decision based on information. As long as you understand the information given to you about your treatment, then consent is deemed to have been given correctly and can be called informed consent. The fact that you sign a piece of paper does not mean you have actually given consent! Education is an important part of the consent process and the piece of paper you sign is only a receipt, with little validity in legal circles. The evidence for consent comes from the records and notes, letters and fact sheets, the drawings and where relevant, models. We act as educators and want you the patient to know as much as possible about the procedure you are signing up to.

Some of this section might seem of little interest, especially if you are familiar with hospitals and treatment centres, or surgery, nurses and activities associated with operating theatres[15] If so, you can skip to the part covering risks.

How did you get to this point?

You started with a painful foot and hopefully have had plenty of opportunity to consider various treatment options and decide what works before considering an invasive method. The pain we know as a neuroma has produced a disability in that you cannot do all that you want to do comfortably. We can measure that disability with a questionnaire[16] breaking down responses into three key elements known as 'domains', each marked out of 100:

- The limits placed on your walking
- Social impact
- Pain

A pathway of care devised by your clinician has guided you through options and stages. You need to decide if you can cope with the condition at this point? Do you want to delay invasive treatment? Have you tried the less well known methods described, and if not, do you want to?

If you feel you have a complete understanding of all that went before and have arrived at the point where you yourself feel surgery could be beneficial, then we need to complete the cycle and deal with consent.

Making a decision

Diagrams, simple drawings and illustrations have been used to help you understand the neuroma condition. While you now know where the incision line will be made, you may still be less aware about after care. What you have not been provided with so far is information about the risks of such surgery. The risks from a general anaesthetic will be discussed by the anaesthetist and are not covered here, but can be found on the RCoA website[14].

Effects of surgery

'I cannot be any worse off than I am now!'

Another misleading quote. Surgery can indeed cause problems.

One patient said that she trusted her clinician even though she did not know all the risks with neuroma surgery. This would be fine until a problem arose and matters changed. Trust is vital, but we need to make sure there can be no lack of understanding. Trust your surgeon but accept all advice given and take it seriously as a problem may happen to you.

Pain at the surgery site may be due to infection pending or poor healing. Too much activity on the foot after surgery will cause swelling[20] and open up the wound. Poor patient compliance implies that the patient has not followed post-operative advice. It is vital to appreciate that not all problems are the foot surgeon's fault; some aspects of care cannot be predicted or prevented.

Where a patient cannot afford time off work or provide total commitment, then it is better to avoid surgery until full compliance can be achieved.

For the most part anything up to an impact factor of 3 (Table 4.1) is generally fully correctable and not unusual. Impact factor 4, however, suggests further treatment or surgery is required and a delay is expected in returning to usual function.

Cysts can arise from skin cells becoming trapped in the wound. Surgery may be warranted because skin repair may become mixed up with suture involvement. It is important to be aware of the low-risk features of a neuroma that have a higher impact.

We can rate consequences or impact following surgery on a scale of 1 to 5 (PASCOM-10)[17,18].

RISKS – BEING AWARE BEFORE THE EVENT

Now that consent has been explained in broad terms you must appreciate the risks that can arise in the context of invasive treatment. Modern surgery limits risk by having a process governed by professional bodies and the World Health Organization we simply now refer to as WHO checks. It should not be possible to reach theatre without numerous checks being made. These may seem tedious but they are designed to protect patients.

Example of questions:

* Has your consent been signed?
* Do you know what you are having done?
* Who will care for you afterwards as you cannot drive? The carer has to be an adult.
* Are you using a taxi or is someone driving you home? Public transport is unacceptable.
* Anaesthetic questions (past experience)
* Has there been any change in your health since last seen?
* Do you have any further questions?
* Has your foot been marked to show the correct site?

RISK LEVEL	EXPECTATION OF EVENT: SEQUELA OR COMPLICATION	FEATURES OF RISK
1	Expected frequently	Features are short-lived and do not involve significant interventions
2	Expected but less frequently	May remain over 3–12 months and then disappear slowly
3	Not expected, but could happen; borderline sequela but complication may arise	May have consequences. Longer treatment times and possible surgery may be required.
4	Not expected, low chance of occurring – always known as a complication	Consequences for function and mobility, some permanent loss possible. Usually containable, but also usually requires further surgery.
5	Difficult to predict, very low likelihood of arising – serious complication	Direct effect on life, possible death, hospitalisation with permanent secondary problems

Table 4.1.

Impact scores for effects of foot surgery[19]

You should NOT sign a consent form if you do not understand what is going to happen after surgery. This means you should fully appreciate that success may vary and that problems might arise that could affect your life.

The easiest way to consider the risks from neuroma surgery is to look at probably the largest U.K foot surgery database from the College of Podiatry (London) foot surgery standing at 95,000 patients *November 2017*. The information in Table 4.2 below comes from a snapshot of the whole of 2016 from 74 centres and covering 944 neuroma treatments, of which 403 (42.7%) confirmed neuroma. The amount of data is helpful to provide a reflection of risk[19].

IMPACT SCORE	PERCENTAGE OF PATIENTS REPORTING	EFFECT
No problems	74.9	Nil
Level 1	2.2	Short-lived
Level 2	8.2	May remain over 3-12 month period
Level 3	11.7	May have consequences with longer treatment period
Level 4	2.9	Usually requires further surgery, function and mobility affected
Level 5	0	Direct negative effect on health for long, indefinite periods

Table 4.2

Neuroma surgery outcome data, 2016

(Source: PASCOM-10)[19]

WHAT TYPE OF PROBLEMS ARISE WITH NEUROMA SURGERY?
In the data provided, out of 403 recorded problems, 302 (74.9%) patients had no ill effects at all. At this point, don't be misled: that means 25% did have a problem of one kind or another. In some patients, surgery was mixed with other operations and so the problems listed may not be specific to the neurectomy procedure alone. The level of impact is shown next to the percentage in Table 4.3

The College of Podiatry uses its database to promote members' contribution to evidence of activity and can be found at www.pascom-10.com, where reports are logged for public view. The data in Tables 4.2 and 4.3 came from a special report on neuroma for this book. It is all well and good having percentage incidences but they do not provide information about impact, i.e., the effect a problem has on an individual. We no longer place an emphasis on

ISSUE OF CONCERN	PERCENTAGE PATIENTS AFFECTED	IMPACT LEVEL
Pain at site of surgery +6 wks.	6.5	3
Scar line raised + or - pain	5	3
Nerve ending scar	2.5	3 or 4
Infection suspected (not proven)	2.0	2
Loss of sensation between toes	1.9	1 or 2
Failed surgery	1.5	4
Delayed wound healing	1.0	3
Blood filled swelling	0.5	3
Patient non-compliance	0.5	3
Large areas of numbness	0.3	3
Complex pain syndrome	0.3	4
Swelling	0.3	1
Skin cyst	0.3	3
Hard skin formation (on sole)	0.3	2
Stitch reaction	0.3	2

Table 4.3

Specific risks with percentage incidence and impact factor. 1 to 4 (0.3 to 6.5% occurrence rate) with low having least effect. The values are taken to one decimal place.

percentage incidences alone, but knowing the chance of something happening is still helpful. If we look at the 15 areas that are common to neuroma we need to consider the impact on a patient. Several problems may need to be bundled together, such as wound healing and infection.

This list in Table 4.3 will not appear on the consent form but will typically shrink down to:

* Blood clot (deep vein thrombosis, DVT)
* Swelling
* Scar problems

* Slow healing
* Possible separation of toes
* Numbness
* Infection
* Complex pain syndrome
* Stiff toes
* Callus formation (if plantar incision made)
* Pain after surgery
* Failure

One caution must be made about impact scores. These have not been tested robustly by scientific method or external review, and more importantly impact scores can vary. The difference between loss of sensation following surgery may be barely perceptible in some cases, and so could rate between 1 (as an expected norm) to 3, based on being unpleasant. The impact score considers the negative effects of surgery affecting patients. Of course, the perception of impact will vary from patient to patient. Note that level 4 concerns may be less frequent but the impact on daily life is greater. This is the best place to start to fully understand your willingness to consent given all information possible.

Local anaesthetic effects
Bruising of the skin or local damage to the nerve can leave the nerve tender for a while until this settles. This probably happens to around 2% of patients. I have seen

one case of extreme sensitivity where the patient had to attend a pain specialist to be injected around the ankle. This may happen in fewer patients, around 0.25%. Skin death from injections is rare but cases do exist and might be related to adrenaline being added to the anaesthetic, causing poor skin healing; adrenaline additives have fallen from favour.

Deep vein thrombosis (DVT)

Blood clot in a vein would feature as a level 3 or 4 concern. To appreciate the risk, we need to look at a larger group of data to see if the incidence rate from a sample of 403 patients was accurate. Taking the period 2010 to mid-2017, 5,331 neurectomy treatments were performed in the UK, and the risk by incidence of DVT was 0.1%, which means a 1 in 1,000 chance.

The impact of having a DVT relates to time to attend and travel to appointments, loss of earnings, worry, cost to healthcare, and the additional risks of using a drug such as warfarin, a blood-thinning drug that needs monitoring. To some patients this may be acceptable but a clot in the leg can lead to chest pain or worse.

Blood-filled swelling (haematoma)
Bacteria are attracted to the swelling, which hardens and the body cannot fight the infection. The foot is painful and may not heal until the hardened blood is removed surgically. Secondary surgery should resolve the problem but adds to overall recovery time (0.1–0.3%).

Nerve scar (nerve stump)
A term that is associated with the end of the cut nerve. The end widens and becomes tethered within the scar. Because the end of the nerve is active, pain from electric shock signals arise. Treatment includes steroid injection initially and then surgical exploration. Electrical destruction (neurolysis) can be used rather than open surgery. The impact is similar to that seen with a DVT except that pain medication may be used longer than usual and can produce side effects (1.0-2.5%).

Healing delay with open wounds
A smaller concern and common for most foot surgery. For neuroma surgery, the incision is small to start with but can easily become infected. The edges of the wound widen slightly. Treatment with antibiotics usually remedies matters, making this an impact level of 2/3. Further surgery can be required, especially where the cause is due to a stitch reaction. This problem arises around 2–3 weeks after surgery (1%).

Splaying of toes

Toes separating is rarely a problem, although may exist before surgery and appear to worsen afterwards.

Sensation loss

As the nerve is cut we can expect to lose sensation. The nerve supplies sensation in the web space: the area shaded in Figure 4.1 represents where this type of problem can occur. There can be sensation loss under the foot as well (0.78–2.0%).

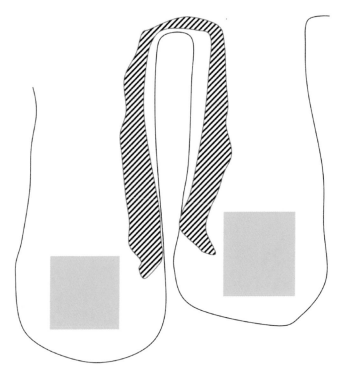

Figure 4.1
Larger areas of sensation loss are rarer and more
likely to be associated with anaesthetic irritation (0.1–
0.25%) around the nerve, which may be bruised.

My story: The impact of sensation loss is acceptable around any wound. In fact, most improve by at least 75%. After my surgery to the left foot, the space between the third and fourth toes was very 'dead'. By six months I had about 15% sensation back, although I felt much better in sandals! This was a local irritation rather than a problem and I would suggest an impact factor of 2. Some numbness appeared under the foot in closed-in shoes – this suggests footwear continues to impact on recovery for much longer than we appreciate.

I did have a patient who was annoyed at me for not informing her that the toe would be numb despite the fact it was mentioned on the consent form. This shows consent forms may not be understood and the information cannot be assured. Larger areas of sensation loss can lead to problems where skin is irritated and the patient cannot sense that damage is being done; this is called neuropathy. As a guide, allow 9–12 months before you can expect nerve sensation to return – and do expect to have a numb toe.

SCARY STUFF

I have not covered every single issue that can arise because some are self-explanatory like swelling. Infection is treated quickly to avoid spreading.

Necrotising fasciitis

This is very rare but can lead to a flesh-eating complication. Bacteria such as streptococci and clostridia rapidly spread and can affect life and limb. Serious infection on a consent form implies necrotising fasciitis but is seldom exaggerated. Necrotising fasciitis comes under impact level 5, i.e., life permanently affected.

Complex regional pain syndrome
Using an analogy of a tap, after surgery pain appears like water dripping out of the tap. The stronger the flow, the worse the pain. With complex regional pain syndrome (CRPS) the tap fails to turn off normally: pain should diminish around 36 hours after a neurectomy and by 72- hours minimal pain should be experienced. Discomfort may continue but should be well controlled by analgesics.

As far as elective neuroma surgery is concerned, nerves are indeed damaged. A nerve stump is minor compared to the increased and constant pain associated with CRPS, which is accompanied by burning. The hot effect causes throbbing and can be unrelenting. The impact factor starts at 3 and at worst can reach 5. The scale varies because some people respond badly and others cope better, but it can take nine months to treat and its emergence may be delayed. Cases reporting at 6–12 weeks are not uncommon. The risk is low at 0.46% but the impact is high. Medication is required and some have side effects. Symptoms of CRPS include:

- Difficulty wearing shoes and walking distances
- Depressed and tearful
- Loss of rationalisation and mood changes

* Occupation and home life can be significantly affected
* Loss of libido or exacerbated erogenous sensitivity

Pain specialists should be consulted early. Further surgery is likely to make matters worse.

SUCCESS AND FAILURE WITH NEURECTOMIES

It is easy to focus on bad things that can happen, but for the most part surgery works well although it is an inconvenient process compared to conservative means. Those who push the methods of cryotherapy and radiofrequency ablation suggest complications are low. In reality all methods have hidden consequences.

Positive outcomes

Outcome is the term we use for the 'end result'. Based on the outcome score called the patient satisfaction questionnaire (PSQ-10) for neuroma, taking a larger group of patients (2,642), an average score of 85.7 was recorded for a longer period than just one year. The higher the value (out of 100) the better the outcome. Looking at the benchmark set by the podiatry profession (that is, a view taken by a panel of experts), the lowest score aimed for would be equal to or greater than 70. In 2016 the data reflected a PSQ-10 score of 87.2, and so the range of expected success for surgery could be expressed as 85.7–87.2. The values shown are the mean or average so a range makes the data clearer. Using 358 completed satisfaction reports, 53.4% scored 91–100. Three patients (0.83%) scored 41–50 and five scored 31–50 (1.3%). This places the chance of complete lack of success at around 0.8–1.5%. However, 88.6% scored higher than the benchmark of 70.

MEETING AIMS – THE CLINICIAN'S TAKE

We all have different interpretations of whether help for the condition we came in for has worked. If it has we can say that the original aim was successful. Nonetheless there is some subjectivity in making that decision. Many patients have more than one problem, which can complicate both the aim and outcome. Where a problem such as Morton's neuroma is isolated, assessing whether our aims have been met is much easier. Where several problems co-exist, the clinician will have to solve all the problems to achieve a good score.

If my patients are better and satisfied, then the aims have been met. I would use the PSQ-10 score to help this judgement, but also the MOXFQ, both of which depend on patient responses. More information about this is covered in Sections 5 and 6.

We break down aims into:

* aims are met   (52%)
* aims are partly met   (7%)
* aims are not met   (0.8%)

The values in brackets highlight the responses by clinicians reflecting their patients' treatment following neuroma surgery. These statistics may look good as we focus on 'aims not met' being low. Of the cases where clinicians recorded data (2,212), 834 did not complete their aims assessment, which translates to 40.2% failed to complete. Clinicians who recorded 'cannot be assessed at this time' imply that mixed problems might have existed to start with and are still being dealt with, or that the patient was undergoing treatment at the time of completing the data. The reasonable interpretation from the data available is that aims are met significantly more times than they are not.

FAILED SURGERY

Failure was recorded as occurring in 1.5% of cases from national data. The reality is that that not all surgery works. What does this mean for the patient? Does the condition become permanent or can it be remedied? What happened to the 11–12% who did not score high?

Achieving reliable data to identify the next part of the journey would be difficult. Failed surgery due to nerve stump pain accounts for the highest amount of recurring symptoms. An association with joint swelling and symptoms around the adjacent joints also can play a part in confusing satisfaction or failing to meet the patient's needs. It is unlikely there will be an absolute state where all surgical intervention works.

SUMMARY

The patient satisfaction score system is sensitive to minor changes, and most patients recover to lead full active lives. Some have complications with an element of impact, and those areas that could affect recovery have been expressed in percentage terms.

Some patients may have had failed surgery because they had multiple conditions and other surgery has affected their end result. The only way to minimise poor outcome is to ensure the diagnosis is as accurate as we can achieve. At this point the truth is that we can give no absolute assurances for neuroma or other conditions associated with the foot.

I would want any patient to take away one key thought.

IMPACT

Surgery has much to offer but there are downsides and patients MUST understand the risks and impact.

- Consent means different things to different people but starts with your initial consultation and ends with your signing a piece of paper called the consent form
- Consent is purely a receipt listing the complications most likely to arise, but it has weaknesses
- The consultation process is never long enough and distractions arise and information can be omitted so always ask: how might a problem affect me?

- Making a decision is based on how your life is affected and the chances of improvement
- Most patients accept these risks but there is no doubt that once they are spelled out some patients are put off and destined not to find a surgical remedy.
- Living with a foot problem is still an option based on patient choice. The only other solution is to ensure that factors causing the problem are omitted as much as possible, e.g., through footwear changes, style of activity and even occupational factors.
- Being forced to change a job you love is not an easy conversation, but one I have had to engage in with an unfortunate few.

I opted for surgery from the top of my foot, and detail my own patient journey in Section 6. In the next section, I will briefly discuss the alternative- surgery from the sole of the foot.

Surgery from the sole of the foot (plantar approach)

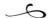

INTRODUCTION

MANY SURGEONS WILL APPROACH THE foot from below because this can offer clearer visibility where the nerve sits under a metatarsal head; from the top the nerve can be obscured. Plantar incisions are also reserved for revision surgery where a nerve is scarred (stump neuroma). I had surgery from the top of my foot (described in Section 6) as did Peter, a hospital colleague, while Brenda and Lisa had surgery from under the foot.

Brenda was a female patient who had surgery from the sole.

CASE STUDY – BRENDA

Brenda was 34 years of age. Her imaging scan from 2014 suggested the diagnosis of a bursa, that is, an organised sac with fluid content inside.

Her steroid injection was no longer helping her and the MOXFQ score before injection recorded: walking comfort value 82; pain 70; and social interference 56. These scores range from 0–100, where low is best.

Naturally the scores were too high. After her injection she was reviewed (at three months) and her new scores showed her walking ability was the same at 82; her pain was down to 60; and her social interference factor was slightly worse at 60. As there was no benefit we discussed the need for a new investigation. As the ultrasound showed the nerve sited under the metatarsal bone, I elected to use an incision under the sole. Her results are shown in Figure 5.1D; the top end of the scar near the toes shows where Brenda has removed some loose skin from a blister. She no longer has pain. This is the desired result from surgery under the sole. Contrast this with Lisa's two-month follow up in

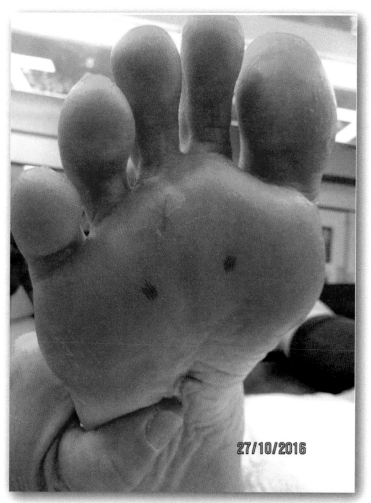

Figure 5.1A
Brenda: pre-operative foot marked carefully
to ensure the incision line falls between the
metatarsal heads marked with black dots.

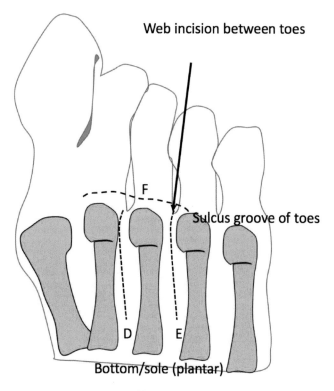

Web incision between toes

F

Sulcus groove of toes

D   E

Bottom/sole (plantar)

Figure 5.1B
Incision sites illustrated under the foot showing
(d) and (e), which are typically used for single
access; F indicates access for both the spaces.

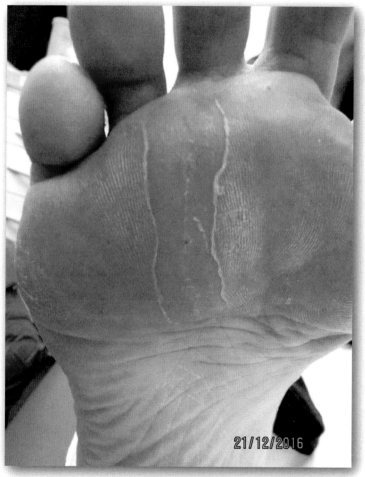

Figure 5.1C
Less than two months later. The skin peels off
and hard skin is more evident at this stage.

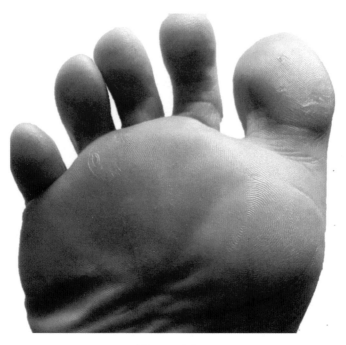

Figure 5.1D
Six months the skin has recovered fully.

POST-OPERATIVE ADVICE

The shift to making an approach from the sole alters recovery slightly, but mainly from the point of view of how much pressure to use. Being unaided (no crutches, no shoes or boot) will hamper mobility and safe movement. The success of surgery still comes down to patients taking care in their recovery and not trying to 'run before they can walk'. Massaging the wound under the sole is very important and can commence once the wound is closed, at around 3–4 weeks. A gel pad would be useful once walking is manageable without aids. The pad will cushion the foot.

Multiple or complex incisions

I have not covered the wider incision under the sole used to remove more than just nerves, but these result in slower recovery than the single incisions shown in Figures 3.2 and 5.1. The general principles remain the same.

RISKS AND AWARENESS

CASE STUDY – LISA

Lisa was 40 when she came to see me for treatment. She had an injection after her ultrasound. Her radiology report could not differentiate between a bursa or neuroma. After little improvement at four months she had surgery under the sole.

The laboratory reported a neuroma. Her stitches came out at just under three weeks. The sole requires stitches to stay in one week longer.

The risks for accessing the nerve from the sole are the same as from the top with one exception: a scar line resting over or near to a metatarsal head can cause pain after the wound has healed.

Corn or callus formation is a thickening of the top skin layer and can develop in or around the scar. We need quite large data samples informing us of this likelihood, but the incidence has been put at 0.35% (sample size of 3,072 patients having neuroma surgery).

The incisions are placed between or above the metatarsals (point F in Figure 3.2), near the sulcus or toe groove.

The risk of scar problems seems low but what of the impact?
Corns are unlikely to resolve, will be permanent and could cause as much pain as before surgery.

Additional surgery to deal with a corn is not easy and many treatment methods fail so in reality a corn is for life. 'Seed corns' are tiny and are better tolerated than deeper corns.

This is what developed on Lisa's sole, as shown in Figure 5.2. The small area of thickening is seen near to the toe end, while the remaining scar line is imperceptible. Once this was scraped away, the underneath looked pink and healthy and was shallow. This could be managed with creams and a pumice stone kept exclusively for her foot. The newer electric roller type shavers appear safe and deal with general hard skin rather than corns.

Lisa no longer has pain and was pleased at this early stage (two months) and awaited her right foot to be operated on; it was equally as painful as the left had been before surgery. Lisa will require occasional podiatry to help her corn.

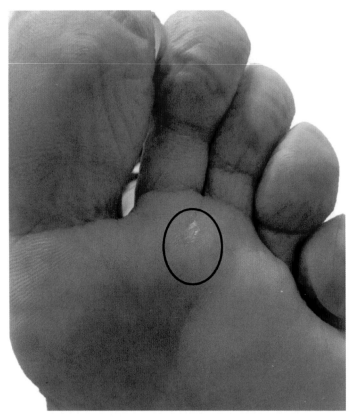

Figure 5.2
Example of seed corn formation encircled with dotted lines

SUMMARY

- Podiatric surgeons use the dorsal approach more frequently
- The use of plantar approach is often down to surgeon preference
- Patients may find the difference and implications useful

The main issues include:

- Longer period of recovery
- Risk of corn formation in the wound
- Scar pain
- Callus formation with ongoing management

On the positive side:

- Nerve access is better
- Valuable with revision surgery
- Potentially lower risk of stump neuroma (Section 4)
- Better access to more than one neuroma

In the next section I will deal with my own journey and experience, but it is essential to point out that this is a single example and others may have different tales.

Planning and what to expect before and after a neurectomy

INTRODUCTION

MOST PATIENTS WILL HAVE INFORMATION provided during their consultation(s) but because of time constraints and pressures placed on clinicians, very few have the luxury of being able to provide all the information possible, and so focus only on the essentials. We rely on patients asking questions to help address specific concerns, otherwise most of us keep to a time-honoured list of pieces of advice.

Leaflets can help, as can the internet. I established my own website in 2013 and populated this with information on every conceivable aspect of surgery relating to my practice. This was updated in 2018 www.consulting-footpain.co.uk and I hope to introduce a new pages in due course.

Producing leaflets causes storage problems, but I like to provide leaflets to direct patients to additional information. While this book is not a leaflet, and runs to more than 25,000 words, most will not read it from cover to cover; it is broken into sections. This is why I have tried to ensure headings and words are highlighted and linked to questions to make navigation easier. The 'whole book' is a resource for reference.

ADMISSION

Surgery commences with admission.

When you arrive at the surgery centre, unit or hospital, more information is provided, but this focuses on recovery, not the operation and risks. It is unlikely that new information will be absorbed when you are sitting/lying on a bed expecting surgery in the next hour or two. Last-minute clarification is about the best you can achieve.

Leaving the unit often catches patients out. Suddenly the surgery is over, they arrive home and at this point wonder, ***'What can I do?'***

Before admission everything seemed reasonable. Numerous information sheets were heaped on the patient. Some of the points missed can include:

- When can I shower?
- How far can I walk?
- Do I really need to take pain medicine?
- When should I start taking the medication?
- How do I climb stairs?
- When can I wear shoes again?

Questions tumble out...

Because we undertake many types of surgery, foot surgeons can often only give broad advice. In this next section I am going to share my own journey[21] after discharge with details of the day-to-day, month-to-month experience. Remember, I know what I have had done, how it was done and know lots about recovery, but even I was surprised by how much I did not know. I have tried to make the narrative interesting as well as informative.

A QUICK REFERENCE TO ADMISSION AND DISCHARGE

Allow time for traffic and check the route to the surgery location the day before and then again on the morning if travelling far.

Admission

- Arrive in good time to avoid being stressed
- Switch your mobile phone off
- Do not take digital photos (there are legal issues here)
- Change into theatre clothing (don't bring personal things to hospital or apply make-up/nail varnish. Leave all valuables at home.
- Check lists and pre-operation information issued (nurse)

- Enter room for anaesthetic administration
- The skin is prepared and cleaned in theatre. The preparation leaves a stain for a little while until full bathing can be engaged.
- A cuff is inflated (ankle or thigh); this stops too much blood obscuring visibility
- The area around the cuff may be slightly tender or ache for a short period
- Surgery is performed and the nerve sample sent for identification
- Into recovery – back to room or ward
- Drink and something to eat
- Information given for discharge, including emergency number and follow-up appointments

Discharge

- What to do at home – rest for first week
- Ensure someone is close to you for at least two days
- Attend clinic for checks with nurse or specialist (on appointment card)
- Sutures taken out unless absorbable
- Skincare of wound (non-greasy products) and massage as directed
- Getting back to shoes 3–6 weeks
- Driving 2–4 weeks depending on manual or automatic car

- Return to work. Pre-plan so as not to overuse the foot. Begin with half-days for the first week.
- Expected full recovery timeline six weeks to six months
- Discharged from care (specific time varies)

MY OWN NINE-MONTH JOURNEY
OPERATION DAY

'Mr Footman' (podiatric surgeon) had a big grin, but was probably more worried than me. Operating on a colleague can't be easy - I know as I have operated on colleagues myself. My pulse and blood pressure were pretty good after the drive and an early rise at 5.45am. Nurse Jean booked me in and I answered a bunch of questions; she merrily ticked off each answer, and ensured I was set up for my consultant to be able to complete the consent started some months before. I opted for surgery from the top of my foot.

'Dr Gasman (anaesthetist) came late, as predicted, and took me through the usual mantra. Am I fit for anaesthetic? Had I starved, did I have allergies and did I take medicines? There is a bit about teeth as some prosthetics are best removed if movable; my false front tooth was secured by a screw so okay. He was happy that I was a good risk. I had had general anaesthetics before, which helped him assess my risk.

Mr Footman had initially been surprised when I asked for general anaesthetic but respected my decision and preference, and was pleased that he could offer this service. I suppose some might ask why? I had had general anaesthetic before and liked the fact that the sleep makes surgery quick and I don't have to watch any fiddling around. It seems pleasant to wake up and it is all done. The other reason, perhaps esoteric in nature to me, was that I do not like the thought of the ankle anaesthetic block, despite the fact that I do this regularly on my own patients. The idea of a sharp electric shock does not appeal. I knew I could also suffer from nerve bruising from the injection, but that was a risk I accepted as rare.

Into the operating theatre...

The blotchy disorientation felt on recovery soon disappeared. The mild sore throat was eased with cold water, then tea and tuna sandwiches as I had of course starved and had had no breakfast.

The 8.00am start was advantageous and we were away by 11.30. My wife appeared and we drove home, a journey of 180 miles. A great service at one of the top units in the UK; no one could complain at that. Nurse Felicity sorted the discharge and made sure I had my pain medicine – this consisted of paracetamol (known as acetaminophen in some countries), separate codeine to be used together with paracetamol if needed, and ibuprofen. Now I do confess to heart burn and take ibuprofen rarely as it upsets my stomach. Providing I use it after food I can get by but I also use a gastric protection drug called omeprazole. She also provided me with a contact number in case of emergencies.

The lack of crutches surprised me[22]; no one gets out of my hospital without those aids. The extent of my numbness made it harder to walk. Mr Footman, like most podiatric surgeons with experience in local anaesthetic, ensures primary pain relief comes from the anaesthetic block. We use the term block as it cuts off all sensation and even pressure is tough to perceive once it reaches its full effect. Without crutches I decided to use my own post-operative cast boot. The shoe provided was great as well but did not afford the same protection or comfort as a boot, especially when outside. The cast boot is called an Aircast™ (Figure 6.1) and makes walking safer, protecting the foot and the wound but also taking pressure away from my surgery site. The contoured sole allowed the foot to roll off without hurting. We lunched at a service station and my wife dropped me off at the entrance while I put on the Aircast. This is where those crutches would have been useful. We were back home by 17.20 and I slid onto the settee and stayed there, leg raised. I used the downstairs bedroom so I could access the walk-in shower room and toilet. Having moved recently and retired, we designed the downstairs as if we were disabled. I was to put all this to the test and was very grateful for our forward planning. My foot was still very numb but I reckoned in a few hours it would be back to normal sensation. I popped my second ibuprofen after food.

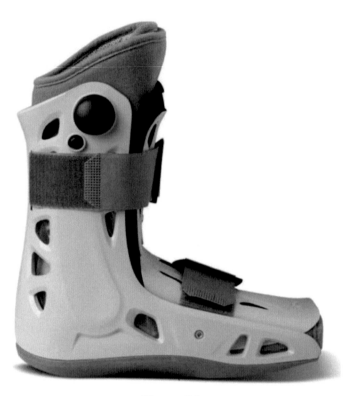

Figure 6.1
The post-operative AircastTM (short boot)

POST SURGERY

Day 1: The anaesthetic block lasted until midnight and then the foot came back to life. That meant it had worked for 15 hours. A forced wiggle (of the foot) brought stinging so I took another ibuprofen despite having loaded myself before sleep with paracetamol and codeine[23]. The wiggle was involuntary and the wound hurt like crazy. My first night had not been so good, but then I don't sleep well anyway. Stinging to throbbing at level 1 using the visual analogue scale in Section 1 (Figure 1.1).

Now the foot sensation was normal, problems with walking became more apparent, but at least it was easier to know how to use my foot without the effects of the anaesthetic and understand how much pressure I could use. Having a full ankle block meant significant heel numbness so I was unsure how much weight my foot would allow against the ground. Of course I had to use the heel in preference to the ball of my foot; that was where my wound was and so needed rest and care. The sole of the foot was definitely uncomfortable so I had to tilt my foot up. This is where I know patients have ankle pain, because the ankle tendons are overused. The post-operative shoe was preferred when getting around without the Aircast, but the Aircast kept the foot better positioned without upsetting my ankle.

A shower was avoided and would have to wait until the initial discomfort eased, allowing me to stand. The sticky dressing was no longer secure and had overlapped.

The foot continued to wax and wane pain wise but standing, of which I did little, always felt better in the Aircast. Hanging the foot down was not too bad. This is a telltale sign as to how things are going: hanging a foot down can be pretty unpleasant in the early days, so I seemed to have overcome the first hurdle in that regard.

My stinging was replaced by throbbing. Paracetamol (x2) 500mg and ibuprofen (x1) 400mg was sufficient to control my discomfort. I avoided the codeine provided knowing that while it was a great pain reliever, it had side effects. The biggest may seem inconsequential, but constipation arises as stool movement is diminished. I used the lower-dose paracetamol (500mg) and codeine (8mg) product Solpadeine, purchased over the counter and dissolved in water for easier swallowing. Constipation is a problem and side effect of codeine as we need normal muscle movement to keep faeces moving. Where constipation is anticipated, drink plenty of water and use laxatives if necessary as discomfort can be unpleasant. Do not use a stronger painkiller than is necessary. Using ice is preferable, but I did not need ice. My second night was much better.

Week 1

Day 2: I had hoped to be further on. Low-grade discomfort around 1-2 mostly 0-1, pain with some discomfort, trickled through my foot. I used my shower cover called a LimbO™cover[24]. No stomach problems fortunately. I rested and used my Aircast for any standing or limited walking. Being able to shower and shave after surgery made me feel human again!

NB. It is important to avoid taping plastic bags around your foot as they will not adequately waterproof the wound. Getting water on the dressing is a sure way of increasing the risk of infection.

Day 3: Better comfort in the night, no extra tablets needed; the stinging sensation lasted five minutes. When walking, the dressing acted like a stone under my foot causing discomfort. I showered comfortably with the LimbO cover; my heel was tender. The reference to my heel was important; I had used the heel when heavily anaesthetised and had favoured this in walking, thinking it made sense without crutches. I now suffered unexpectedly. Because information was not getting to my brain when the foot was anaesthetised, I could not control the pressure applied and the heel soon became bruised with 11.5 stone (73 Kg) loading it. Again the Aircast helped enormously. I found some crutches as well so thankfully I had all the aids required.

Day 4: Pain was now around 0 unless I stretched my foot out – then the wound hurt like mad. Walking was difficult. I stripped down the wound and found the skin bruised and tender. This was normal and as I would see in my own patients. Bruises around the heel and away from the wound were common. I applied my own light dressing to replace the one provided. There was minimal bleeding so the risk of a blood-filled swelling was now unlikely. I could see the ends of the sutures. Mr Footman had used dissolvable stitches, which meant only the ends would need trimming, but I could get my own nurses to do that at two weeks. Bruising on the second toe was notable but again no more than I would have expected. Feeling something strange under my foot correlated to patient reports but otherwise I felt fine. I had an appointment at the dentist but got there without too much problem using crutches and boots and being driven to the door.

WEEK 2

Day 7: I left my dressing off for the first time after my shower. The 'rucked-up sock' feeling persisted, even in my boot. Twinges still arose but I needed no pain control. My car was an automatic so I could drive and was back at work for one day only. My nurses were brilliant and brought patients down, saving me walking. All had been briefed and asked how I was doing. It is curious being in the health market where everyone was keen to know how it went. Patients asked – 'Did you do the surgery yourself? Meanwhile the boot was a helpful discussion point with patients coming in expecting surgery.

Day 8: The foot – yep, swollen, and hurt toward the end of the evening, looking a bit like a balloon compared to normal. I resisted an ibuprofen but got into bed early feeling fairly tired. This was a non-compliance issue to be honest: I should have cancelled all commitments or gone back to work for only half a day. Even the surgeon failed to take his own advice!

Day 9: Bruising was still present and the cast boot felt loose. The front piece was important now to keep the boot comfortable. Tubigrip™ provided by my hospital helped as an extra sock. I removed the dressing and decided to leave the wound to dry out. This turned out to be a positive experience as the wound was ready to be left open. I would normally keep dressings[25] on patients for longer.

Day 10: By now I could fully weight bear. Tender sensations existed and the fullness (bursting effect) under my foot had ceased. I was still showering with the LimbO cover. The skin was settling and had lost its redness. Sensations of soreness, pulling and rubbing all came and went. Some of the old sticky tape residue remained as the foot could not be immersed fully in water.

Day 11: Foot pressure was better tolerated. Occasional uncomfortable twinges, even burning arose momentarily. The slinky stitches shone where light caught the loops at the end of the wound. The wound was calmer and sandals proved the best footwear, provided the adjustable front strap did not rub if too tight. I stuck with these.

Day 12: Sandals did seem helpful but the straps needed padding (I used felt) to keep the front away from the foot. However, it was too soon for (closed in) shoes. The bruising slowly disappeared and the contact sensation, while still uncomfortable, was unpleasant more than painful. Burning occurred at rest but was fleeting. Aching is the best description, and only when the foot was stressed, but the numbness was notable where the nerve was removed between the toes. Swelling was controlled now as I was more careful in not overusing the foot. I made sure I sat rather than stood and kept the foot and leg elevated.

Day 13: The foot started stinging when I rolled over on the operation side at bedtime. The sensation underneath was clearly abnormal! The numbness confuses the brain and it feels as if a lump is still present, even though there is nothing under the foot. My nerves were overactive and sending weird messages. Walking with sandals was quite tolerable, but increasing my walking distance was less comfortable. The incision could now be touched nearest the ankle end, otherwise there was some redness. This might have been caused by the sandal buckle compressing the skin slightly. Foot swelling was now minimal and general foot colour[26] good.

WEEK 3

Day 14: A nurse colleague trimmed the stitches, cutting the loops flush, pulling a little as she went. The slight soreness stopped after a few moments. I spotted that the middle of the wound had healed and the end was a little scabby. It was now comfortable enough to switch back to using my closed-in shoes rather than sandals. What was that lump? The shoe was flat inside. The sensation yet again broke through, uncomfortable, occasionally sore rather than painful. I was limping, trying to make the best of it. I was back at work now, but only for three half-days.

Day 15: The foot was stingy after walking in town; maybe half a mile. I started creaming the scar and made a greater effort at massage. I noted a funny sensation like an electric shock under the foot. As expected the deep pressure caused tenderness as the scars in the soft tissue were still settling. Another pair of shoes proved more comfortable than my work shoes. Walking slowed down to compensate; for once I walked more slowly than my wife!

Day 16: Driving and minimal walking was otherwise going well. Furthermore, my foot felt better for the rest and light use, but I became aware that the fourth toe had a mild sting. Itching came and went. I wanted to keep the foot cool as this was more comfortable.

Day 17: On massaging the foot in the evening I noticed the scab was still thick at one end. Some inflammation was present in the form of a deeper red colour, but the centre of the scar was flat and had mostly healed.

Days 18–20: The benefit from surgery was now evident save for the definite lumpy sensation when walking.

There was a burning sensation around the fourth toe. I massaged the scar lightly after my shower to ease away the scabs present. The central scar was soft. Foot massage caused nerve end irritation. A deep, aching pain sensation arose for a short spell, but this was wholly expected. I wondered if this was a stump neuroma, so I massaged all the harder. Walking felt as if there was a stone in even my most comfortable shoes. The scabs at both ends of the scar were still stubborn. I noticed the nerve around my ankle where I was injected was achy. This would be a tick for one of those minor complications – impact level =1

Week 4

Day 21: The scab at the toe end finally peeled away in the shower (see Figure 6.2), but pain gnawed down my fourth toe as I massaged. It was as if the loss of sensation was replaced with deeper nerve activity. Directing my massage to the sole, the nerve flickered uncomfortably as if still present. A general achy tenderness existed around the operation site, but there was no swelling. Walking was uncomfortable; the pad of the foot felt as if a wad of sock was rucked up. Later that day a sharp shooting electric shock into the fourth toe kept occurring as I was driving – enough to keep me alert when the waves came. These bursts lasted 5–10 seconds at most. I was driving an automatic for my left operated foot.

Days 23–26: When my foot hit the ground first thing in the morning I noted soreness but the strange sensation wore off after a few steps. I dried in between toes carefully and noted the numbness; strange but not unpleasant. At the end of the day, I noted that my foot ached with a soreness I had not experienced, intermingled with a sensation of itching. The scar was changing colour and looked more like a healed incision line now at just over three weeks. My foot was noticeably tender over the fourth/fifth nail. I tried cutting it back and there was no problem with length or thickness. The changes in nerve messages seemed disturbed and occasionally I could feel intense discomfort. This was something I had been unaware of as a foot surgeon, but now when I talk to patients, the sensation of a nail being sensitive is not uncommon.

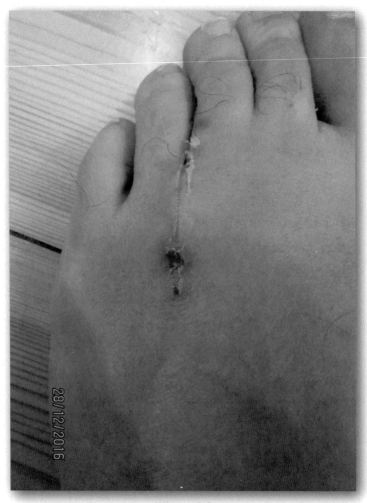

Figure 6.2
Wound on top of the foot at 21 days. The end
furthest from the toe remains unhealed

An anti-inflammatory tablet helped my foot during the night but the mild form of nerve pain was part of normal recovery. I managed a walk down the road to the end and back in my boots (0.7 mile). It was progress, although the top of the foot was uncomfortable at times, as if a needle had been stuck in me where it ached. The scab stood out as the darker colour faded elsewhere. Overall though – progress!

Days 27–30: Walking was slowly easier but that lump sensation moved sideways. I was back working in theatre operating without any problems and my theatre clogs were comfortable.

Furthermore, in clinic I could easily manage to collect my own patients. By Day 30 my foot behaved and was comfortable in my ankle boot. This was the first time I felt the day went well with the foot in mind.

So, we can say at this point that the idea of a four-week recovery is fairly accurate.

MONTH 2

Day 31: I celebrated today after doing a four-mile cycle ride in soft shoes. The foot remained comfortable and did not show any ill effects except some aching. The increased sensitivity seemed manageable. This was a breakthrough now at four weeks and three days and brought a sense of achievement.

Day 34: The gel pad I had ordered worked well once the odd feeling dispersed. The gel pad is also helpful for scar lines on the sole of the foot; however, it did not fit all my shoes. It seems that sensations vary from day to day and each one creates a new experience, but these were only minor concerns and one soon adjusted each time.

Days 37–38: More activity now: I walked down the lane, the January air was cool but pleasant. In walking boots the new pad managed well enough and was comfortable most of the time. The toe made a shooting sensation but otherwise seemed fine. That scab was still in place (Figure 6.2). Most of the limp was now minimal and I was cycling up to 16 miles with my official cycle shoes. The last scab finally came away during the day, leaving a blemish on the otherwise finer linear scar line (Figure 6.3).

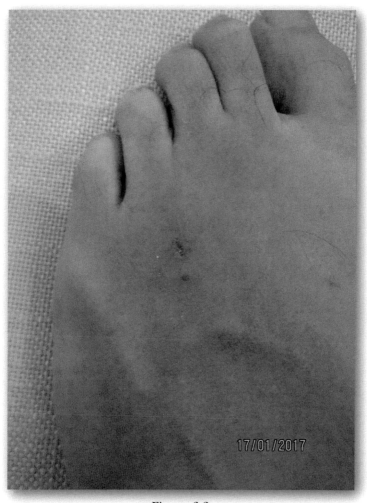

Figure 6.3
Wound on top of the foot at 38 days. The end
furthest from the toe has healed but has been
irritated and delayed because of stitch reaction.
This is common to feet and often unreported

Contrasting with the advice I give to patients, recovery at 4–6 weeks seemed reasonable, and I now looked toward the second milestone: three months to lose the 'cotton wool' effect under the sole. This did not usually cause tenderness but was just an annoyance I could ignore for the most part. For women – shoe design selection would be far more important. The top of the foot could rub and inevitably leave soreness upon shoe removal. Following a two-mile walk I realised it would not be the walking I had to monitor: six weeks of no exercise had led to some weight gain, which was another challenge to overcome.

Days 40–58: That first morning step still sent out messages, the sensation dense and unpleasant, not painful but adjacent to where the neuroma was. Again confusion of messages to and from this small digital nerve. When I poked my foot the tenderness had diminished and walking continued to improve when visiting town. The scar line had settled well; a faint line and no colour changes of concern. The air temperature remained cold at around zero. A bout of spasm was experienced in bed, the first so far. Was the numbness just a little less?

At nearly eight weeks, an uncomfortable pressure sensation still existed during that first step out of bed. The bustle of the day removed most sensations. On Day 58 I was away on holiday and booked in for a massage – the masseur did a good job. I was apprehensive as she massaged the sole but it turned out okay.

MONTH 3

Day 68: My foot had healed well enough and I was accustomed to my new numbness. Different styles of shoes made a difference; sandals and Crocs were the least troublesome. Semi-unpleasant sensations could still break through consciousness.

Day 78: Mr Footman asked about my progress via email. I responded:

'Doing well enough, but the sole shows signs of numbness in a different way and I will await the three-month and nine-month marks for nerve restoration or not. Walking bare foot is strange, but not troubled too much, or when walking on sand. But the sensation is something one could not exclude, even though not uncomfortable.'

MONTH 4

Day 97: I looked at my foot, as I did so often. The incision line had a blemish, assumed to be permanent. The lack of sensation was still profound. Walking had normalised; having acclimatised I had little discomfort in the sense of abnormal fullness. The wound on top of the foot was not sensitive but retained some light yet tolerable tender sensations.

So there I was 13 weeks down the line and you could say this fitted with my own prediction of a three-month recovery. Nonetheless I was still surprised at the length of time and impact on walking.

Month 5

Day 143: Back out on my bike for a short cycle of seven miles in misty fog. The foot was desperately numb – too much compression (from the shoe and thicker sock). No pain but a strange sensation that lasted into the next day. My first setback.

Month 6

This is the ideal period of time lapse to assess the success of surgery. Improvement is still expected and the full recovery will take up to one year. I experienced sensations under my foot still in some, but not all, shoes.

Month 9

The period when we as professionals say nerve sensation usually returns. The bottom of my foot now has a strange sensation that cannot be described as painful but it is a departure from normal. One side of the toe is duller than the other, but on the whole better with signs of improvement. On a few occasions a sharp, well-focused pain radiates into the end of my toe. It hurts (visual analogue scale = 3) but lasts under two minutes. I still get some spasms. Closed-in shoes are always more sensitive than open toe sandals. Can I get used to this? Yes, the foot is better now compared with the discomfort I had before surgery, which was unpredictable. I might have weird sensations but I can live with these and they are predictable. I do have an occasional suggestion of burning, but this is marginal. I know many of my own patients do not have similar features while others do. Taking a cross section, the end result clearly varies.

I recorded the clinical value based on before- and after-surgery MOXFQ and patient satisfaction score, shown in Table 6.1:

SATISFACTION	SCORE 93
OVERALL IMPROVEMENT	91%
walking and standing ability	100%
social interaction	84%
pain	91%

Table 6.1

Clinical assessment of my own results using questionnaire tools. Social interaction is coping with everyday mobility

WHAT TO LOOK FOR IN AN INFECTION?

- Usually arises after 48 hours and notable if pain management is no longer controlled
- Pain may become uncontrolled at rest, swelling arises with significant increased tenderness
- The foot may feel as if it is 'bursting'
- Skin colour darkens and spreads toward the ankle
- The wound may burst open and bleed or show heavy discharge
- Sleep is affected and if serious patients become unwell fast
- Appetite loss, may have diarrhea, and vomit
- Core temperature rises above 36.7° C

The latter signs require urgent management and can require overnight admission to hospital

Conclusion

I am no longer affected at work or at home, and reflect on my patients who consult me for this problem. Maybe I can confess to being a true expert now? Perhaps I am more frank with patients than I once was, reflecting on an experience I want to share.

Claudia was around my age and returned at two months. This was the usual discharge point after surgery.

'Will it get any better?'

Reassurance is important, but there is that lingering unknown about just how much sensation loss will arise. I tell her she still has some time ahead before we can make that judgement. Claudia is a gardener and can return to work. I sent her off with the usual paperwork, which once completed will provide me with those scores I like to collect.

Summary

I recognised that I had swapped one set of sensations for another. We (as patients) must appreciate that we can rarely return exactly to where we were before our symptoms arose.

- Neuroma surgery can be performed under local or general anaesthesia as day surgery

- Swelling will arise if not rested (10 days' essential rest)
- The first night's sleep after neurectomy can be poor but not necessarily painful
- If taking codeine you may need to use a laxative and should drink at least one litre of water per day
- The first week you will need plenty of rest. Crutches or an Aircast™ type design boot are valuable for neuroma. A post-operative shoe would be a minimum expectation.
- Rest includes elevation of the leg and careful use of pain medication to avoid constipation or stomach upset, but do take when needed
- Bathing okay by Day 2/3 with shower cover (LimbO™ cover)
- Dressing can be left off if the wound is stable (ask). Will dry faster if open.
- Walking around is okay, protection important
- Return to shoes by six weeks
- You should be able to return to work after 2-3 weeks, but start slowly, with half days
- The wound may retain scabbing for six weeks
- Start massaging the foot at three weeks
- The lumpy/cotton wool effect diminishes by six months
- Numbness might still be present at nine months

- Localised sensation loss under the foot may be permanent
- Sharp pain at the end of the toe lasts moments

I expect to improve but most of the healing has been completed.

The skin heals quickly but may have some longer-term discolouration.

My operation was successful because it met my aims, which was to be free of pain. Final thoughts are recorded in the last section.

SECTION 7

Final thoughts and loose ends

INTRODUCTION

I HAVE TRIED TO SET out my thoughts on treatment with a strong emphasis on experience across a wide spectrum. Success can only be established when the condition can be arrested early in the day. The spectrum covers self-help – conservative treatment, steroid injections and finally surgery. I have shown how the dedicated profession of podiatry and its surgical wing, podiatric surgery, has considered evidence of effectiveness and emphasised concerns for risk and impact.

At the time of writing we have collected over 90,000 patient care episodes. No foot surgeon likes problems or unhappy patients, but we do accept that problems arise. Those that relate to impact levels 1–3 are usually satisfactory, if not inconvenient, and the patient satisfaction score (a separate measure) tends to point to this when it is above 60. A low score of 30–50 usually means the patient is unhappy and naturally we should do all we can to avoid poor satisfaction. It is difficult to achieve 100% improvement for everyone and whilst ideal as a bench-mark[27], this cannot be assured. The reason for this will be elaborated later in this section.

FACTORS THAT MAKE SURGERY SUCCESSFUL

It is a fact that if the patient and the clinician are both pleased with the results from treatment then the aims have been met. Where the patient alone is pleased the same generally applies, but not the other way around, even if it was the most brilliant surgery. Fortunately, this happens rarely.

I would like to share with you how we view our patient satisfaction. My own satisfaction was rated at 93 marks. We avoid calling this a percentage because the score is affected by a range of different factors that depend on the type of surgery, e.g., how long it takes to return to footwear; bunion surgery takes longer to recover from than an ingrowing toe nail, for example.

To decide if patients are happy we use criteria to weight each question. Were the original expectations (considered before treatment) met? This telltale question punches above its weight when compared to other questions. For neuroma surgery the data taken from 2010–2017 (5,331 patient treatments) delivered 2,642 responses, a return of just under 50% (which is excellent by comparison with most questionnaires). The average reported satisfaction score was 85.7, so well above the benchmark of 70.

Twenty-two percent had minor problems after surgery, but only 2.3% had a major problem. We will assume that 'minor' relates to an impact level of ≤3 and major, 3–4. We know that there have been no level 5s reported to date.

Return to footwear is defined as being able to use closed-in shoes rather than sandals. Typically, 85% of patients are back in shoes by eight weeks, with 50% back by four weeks. I returned to shoes within three weeks.

In terms of the original problem we asked if patients were better or worse: 88% were either better or much better, with 92.3% suggesting they would have surgery under the same circumstances again.

Seventy-nine percent indicated that their aims were met and only 4.5% that their aims were not met. Fifteen percent felt they had their objectives met in part, which meant that other foot problems probably co-existed. Nearly 2% said that they had deteriorated (after surgery) and 3% were a little worse. Nearly 6% indicated they were the same and 1.2% failed to answer the question.

Being better is neither black nor white. One of the key questions that makes up the satisfaction score covers discomfort from the original problem at six months. The worst outcome is that pain still arises at rest. In our survey of 2,642 responses, 10.6% had pain at rest compared to 5.6% when standing, or for longer periods of standing

13.1%. The occasional twinge reflected my own experience and was responsible for dropping my score from 100 to 93. This means the score system is sensitive and if I had known this (the system scores the respondents blindly) I could have fudged it to give my colleague a better reference. It turned out that I was amongst the 41.7% who had this occasional twinge! For neuroma surgery this seems normal. Complete absence of discomfort was reported in only 27.7%, although 1.3% did not respond.

I wanted to reflect my male colleague's experience as he also had surgery approached from the top while my patient Brenda had surgery under the foot. Peter did better than me at 98 (Table 7.1). The values vary but all show overall improvement. As a foot surgeon I have learned so much from writing up my own journey and now stride to make improvements by educating patients – and maybe colleagues?

Post-surgery evaluation	Peter Top incision	Me Top incision	Brenda Bottom incision
SATISFACTION	98	93	93
OVERALL IMPROVEMENT	90%	91%	91%
walking and standing ability	100%	100%	96%
social interaction	100%	84%	100%
pain	85%	91%	75%

Table 7.1

Contrasting three cases at six months post neuroma surgery

FINAL ANALYSIS

A neuroma does not come overnight but arises slowly, and the patient, usually a female over 40 years of age, only notices symptoms when the regularity increases. I was around 56 when my symptoms probably started. It can take up to two years to become aware that you have a neuroma; beyond this the nerve sheath may already have been damaged and so reversal is unlikely to be possible. The schematic illustration in Figure 7.3 is an impression based on my clinical experience both as a surgeon and as a patient.

ORTHOTIC INLAYS AND STEROID INJECTIONS

The orthotic inlay worked well but I left the steroid injection too long and wished I had tried this sooner. Every time the orthotic was used symptoms would drop by 70–95%, so I became used to accepting the condition as it was controlled. Spasms of my muscles increased and

Timeline – the neuroma

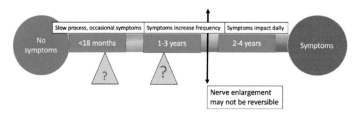

Figure 7.1
Neuroma timeline: A lag period is likely to exist
before we seek help. The golden period of opportunity
lies within the first 18 months perhaps?

affected me particularly at night in bed – I had to get up and walk to break the spasm. By the time I started to increase cycling and use narrower shoes, the symptoms peaked again, leaving me with distinct numbness. This was when an injection was used and failed. This told me that my nerve had been damaged irreversibly.

Mr Footman took the nerve out and thought it very large. The moral to the tale is YES, we can do something much earlier, but we have to take control and not ignore those telltale symptoms.

Shooting pain, on and off pain, or pain anywhere around the toes causing changes in sensation. It may be too late to reverse the damage by this stage, but don't give up.

OPTING FOR SURGERY

The operation worked for me but I believe that the effect leaves lifelong changes that you have to be prepared for. Numbness is not a big issue, perhaps an irritant at most. Colour changes will disappear and massage is essential from Week 3 onwards. Don't go back to work too soon. Two weeks is probably about right, not 1 week like I did. Expect swelling for a while and if you have dogs to walk (we have a cat) then get someone else to walk man's best friend. The wound is all important and you must take care of it at all costs.

Should we go top or bottom of the foot?

Podiatrists seem to advocate the top of the foot approach (Points B or C in Figure 3.2). When reviewing data 10 out of 11 cases (91%) were operated from the top.

With more information hopefully you can speak more confidently to your foot surgeon, although I would not advocate using my book other than for a calm discussion. We all have strong views. I elected for the bottom of the foot approach for Brenda and Lisa. When operating on two neuromata I prefer the sulcal approach although I have also operated from the top. I just don't like to take unnecessary risks. Sometimes there is little choice. I would say possibly the biggest plus for the top is faster recovery as it appears less post-operative skin care is needed. The biggest pluses for underneath are better access, reduced chance of a stump neuroma and maybe also of failure.

QUICK CHECK LIST	TOP	BOTTOM
Scar visible	x	
Scar likely to form a corn		
Possible numbness in toe	x	
Reduced risk of stump neuroma		x
Shorter recovery (about 1-3 weeks)	x	

Table 7.2

Top or bottom approach pros and cons This may be deceptive, as both incision approaches have different benefits positive choice.

Conclusion

I hope this book has provided you with useful insight into the world of foot pain and Morton's neuroma. While scientific analysis is critical to justify comments, much of this book comes from field experience and may be more realistic than scientific papers. Nonetheless I have used some good old-fashioned audit data to offer a realistic view and snapshot of the effects of neuroma treatment.

Fact sheets may be all you need, but such sheets distil many points, leaving unanswered questions. The internet is a valuable resource but bear in mind it carries massive advertising potential for products and promises, and that you need to filter out unreliable or even misleading information.

Professional websites are useful. Those with an academic interest should seek out professional papers from the UK such as in The Foot and The Journal of Foot and

Ankle Research (JFAR). From the United States, Foot and Ankle International and The Journal of Foot and Ankle Surgery. Other journals and periodicals exist, though some are not specific to the foot and ankle. Local libraries, the British lending library and internet searches may prove helpful, and are free of charge.

I hope the journey I experienced and described will better prepare you if you need surgery. Of course if you are in the process of recovering, the points I make may still be helpful and reassuring. If you know someone who has symptoms similar to yours then consider recommending my book on the patient's journey. Thanks for reading this book. Please use it as a guide, a fill in, but not as a dogmatic statement of musts. Remember you want to remain on good terms with your specialist, after all.

If you are willing to provide a review and rate this book your feedback will help others.

Good luck!

Professionals

1. The College of Podiatry is part of The Society of Chiropodists & Podiatrists: www.feetforlife.org.

2. The relevant subgroup of the British Orthopaedic Association is called the British Orthopaedic Foot and Ankle Society: http://www.bofas.org.uk/

3. The main professional body is The Society of Chiropodists & Podiatrists. All podiatrists have to be registered in UK law under the Health Care Professions Council (HCPC): http://www.hpc-uk. org/to use the title podiatrist and are independent of the medical colleges.

Section 1

4. **Aims and outcome** for foot surgery were described by Tollafield & Parmar in 1992 as part of a patient audit project initially using 112 patients at the University of Northampton.

5. **Podiatry professionals** working in the independent sector will make a charge. Patients may use a named healthcare provider often referred to as medically insured or may pay for care themselves. Small health savings funds, where regular payments are made

toward that, may pay for consultations or treatment. Always check who is covered.

6. The **regulator** is a body of people made up of a mix of healthcare professionals and lay people, usually approved by The Secretary of State for Health in the UK. Professionals retain their licence to practice as part of a cyclical process and complaints from the public are upheld where appropriate. Hearings are similar to law courts with lawyers supporting the process. Assessment of a professional person's practice is regularly reviewed by the regulator.

Section 2

7. **Thomas Morton** described the feature of his neuroma in 1876, although British chiropodist Lewis Durlacher wrote about the condition in 1845. Morton, from the USA, managed to publish to a wider audience and thus bestowed his name on the neuroma.

8. **Malignancy** in feet is rare. As a primary diagnosis I have seen only five proven malignancies in a 40-year career. Clinically we always sample tissue to check something is not missed. Accuracy can be improved by using tests such as MRI and ultrasound, giving around 95% assurance. Symptoms that mimic neuroma turn the surgery into an exploratory procedure.

Before we had ultrasound, operations without finding a neuroma could lead to disappointment.

9. **Bleeding and scarring.** Any bleeding in body tissue forms a clot; a hardened mass is replaced by scar tissue. Scars are formed from fibres of collagen. Where this is unhelpful we use the term fibrosis, a disruptive condition of fibre caused by over-management by the body around the nerve.

Section 3

10. **Reflexology**, also known as zone therapy, is an <u>alternative medicine</u> involving the <u>application of pressure</u> to the feet and hands with specific thumb, finger and hand techniques without the use of oils or lotions. It is based on a pseudoscientific system of zones and reflex areas that purportedly reflect an image of the body on the feet and hands, with the premise that such work effects a physical change to the body. There is no convincing evidence that reflexology is effective for any medical condition: https://en.wikipedia.org/wiki/Reflexology

11. **British Acupuncture Council**: 'Treatment involves the insertion of very fine needles into specific points on the body to affect the flow of your body's qi, or vital energy.' :www.acupuncture.org.uk

12. **Homeopathy** is a natural form of medicine used by over 200 million people worldwide to treat both acute and chronic conditions. It is based on the principle of 'like cures like'. In other words, a substance taken in small amounts will cure the same symptoms it causes if taken in large amounts: www.britishhomeopathic.org

13. It is easy to be hoodwinked by **data**. Attitude to the size of data is topical. Larger numbers drawn from a population sample help the overall picture. Compare this to an election poll. Small numbers do not represent large communities accurately. The sciences of data (statistics and epidemiology) are outside the remit of this book, however.

14. For more information, the **Royal College of Anaesthetists** (RCoA) provides a useful website: rcoa.ac.uk – look for 'Patient and Carers on the top menu band and click: http://www.rcoa.ac.uk/

Section 4

15. In the USA **operating theatres** are called operating rooms or OR. British medicine used the word theatre due to historical lineage from public amphitheatre displays.

16. The **questionnaire** is called the Manchester-Oxford Foot Questionnaire or MOXFQ, and was originally designed specifically for bunion surgery effectiveness. The questionnaire has been found to be valuable for a wide range of foot surgeries. Each domain is marked by a computer to find an overall score 0-100, where 0 is excellent and 100 is the worst score.

17. **Evidence** - Impact scores were designed as part of the PASCOM-10 database and audit tool and promoted as Negative Performance Indicators initially. The latest version is found within PASCOM-10 Invasive Domain Guide User Guide, version 1.04; December 2014. © College of Podiatry: www.pascom-10.com

18. **Data** were provided with permission from the Chair of the PASCOM-10 working party, September 2017.

19. Unless stated all podiatric patient data is taken from the period January 2010-June 2017: www.pascom-10.com. This report has only been published internally.

20. **Swelling** may or may not be a complication but simple swelling is probably a little more common than the data suggest. In the majority of cases swelling should be minimal by four months.

Section 6

21. This **journey** was taken from a contemporaneous diary. The original present tense has been changed to past tense. Such detail cannot be achieved by recall.

22. It is important to recognise that I was travelling a long distance back home, and for patients living closer to the unit, crutches may not always be issued. My comments do not reflect any omission of care received. The decision to use a centre so far away from home was my choice.

23. **Pain killer – codeine**. I know as a clinician that preventative pain care is important so that sleep is not broken. Sleep is vital for recovery, preventing the foot from hurting reduces the chance of a rude awakening.

24. The **LimbO™ cover** is a reinforced plastic jacket that has a neoprene rubber gasket to prevent water entering. It is designed for recovery, and used for all patients after surgery as allowing showers is important: https://limboproducts.co.uk/product/limbo-foot-cover-m20

25. **Dressing** for covering wounds after surgery always creates a debate. Any decision must consider the state

of the wound after neuroma surgery, its location and clinician preference. Not all wounds can be left open, especially if there is some ooze or bleeding.

26. **Colour of the foot.** After surgery patients can expect the foot to have a deep red or even purple colour, which settles usually by six weeks.

Section 7

27. **Benchmark** is a term that places a value considered reasonable to achieve for treatment. We set our benchmark based on earlier studies at 70. Seven-year follow-up studies have been used to show the effect of this value over time. The majority of satisfaction values for neuroma surgery are greater than 70.

GLOSSARY OF TERMINOLOGY

Although the language used has been simplified, in some places 'medical' terminology is necessary.

Admission
A process of taking a patient into a care unit (day) or hospital for treatment. The opposite is *discharge*, leaving a care unit or hospital after treatment

Anaesthetic
A chemical agent that can remove pain and induce sleep. Most frequently prefixed by *local*. Local anaesthetic only removes pain and is also called a local analgesic.

Analgesic
A chemical or therapeutic agent used on the skin or taken by some other route, usually by mouth that can provide pain relief, e.g paracetamol and codeine

Anti-inflammatory
An agent that interfers with the process of inflammation helpful in reducing pain e.g ibuprofen (pronounced *eye-bew-pro-fen*)

Bursa
Organised sac provides cushion between a hard and soft structure, sometimes found normally but can become inflamed as in *metatarsalgia*

Chiropodist

Old term still in use today but no longer a formal qualification and was replaced around 1988 with new University degree courses in Podiatry.

Cryosurgery

The application of a gas or liquid that has the ability to freeze tissue below a point where human cells can normally survive. Also see cryotherapy.

Cryotherapy

Any treatment that uses cold e.g ice packs.

Data

Information gathered from a patient that can be analysed into meaningful information. It may be stored on paper or within a computer system. Strict rules govern the use and storage of health data.

Day care unit

A purpose built area in a hospital or health centre usually with the intention of providing surgery which does not require the need for admission overnight.

Diastasis

Separation of toes where they would normally be closer.

Flare-up
Unexpected inflammatory reaction (as in short lived steroid side effect).

Hypersensitivity
A point at which the skin (more often) reacts to light touch in such a manner that the sensation is unpleasant.

Interossei
Small strap like muscles between metatarsals with weak movement effect on toes.

Lesion
Term used to indicate any abnormal change in connective tissue cells; skin, bone, joint, nerve.

Metatarsalgia
Associated with any pain under the ball of the foot (heads of metatarsals).

Metatarsal
Five long bones in the foot which join to toes.

Paraesthesiae
'Pins and needles' forming an abnormal sensation when a nerve is stimulated. Example irritation around nerve around elbow gives 'funny elbow' symptoms shoot down the arm into fingers.

Sclerosing agent
Usually an injectable substance that causes hardening of connective tissue

Suture
Means 'seam'. Material used to close a skin defect that would otherwise be slow to heal under normal circumstances. The same as 'stitch'.

Synovitis
Inflamed joint lining.

White blood cells
Special defensive cells produced and will increase in numbers to act against any harmful agent whether chemical or infective often creating pus as part of the reaction.

'Progress through the art of communication'™ © **2015**

Look out for more foot journey books from David
Tollafield during 2018-19

Follow him on Likedin, twitter and Facebook

Also

Website Consultingfootpain.co.uk
with blogs on *Footlocker*

e-mail: myfootjourneys@mail.com

Made in the USA
Coppell, TX
03 July 2022

79520768R10117